CLOSE-UP

WINNING THE AGE GAME
NEW BEGINNINGS:
COSMETIC SURGERY FOR MEN AND WOMEN

CLOSE-UP

Gloria Heidi's
10-Day Makeover Program

ILLUSTRATIONS BY MARK CHIARELLO

G. P. PUTNAM'S SONS
NEW YORK

Photographs courtesy of Clairol

Library of Congress Cataloging in Publication Data

Heidi, Gloria.
Close-up: Gloria Heidi's 10-day makeover program.

1. Beauty, Personal.   I.   Title.
RA778.H446   1984   646.7'042   84-8230
ISBN 0-399-12979-0

Printed in the United States of America

Designed by Lynn Braswell

Contents

CLOSE-UP

Peter Marshall and I make a Cinderella fantasy come true on NBC's "Fantasy."

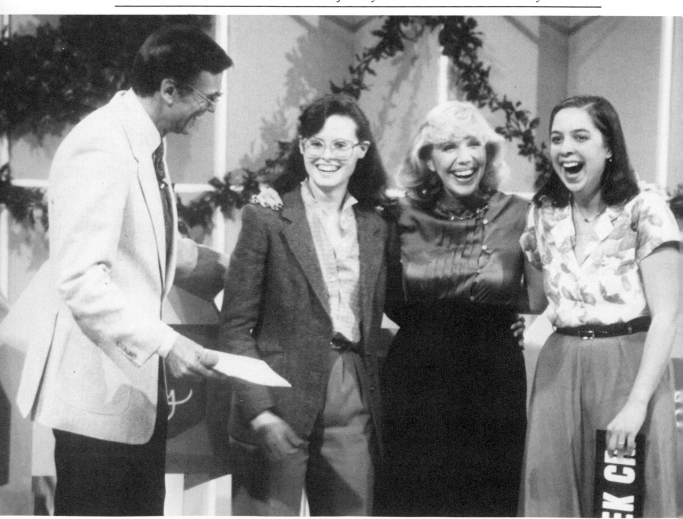

One

Today Is the Day

"This makeover is the most wonderful thing that's ever happened to me!"

"I never dreamed I could look and feel this terrific!"

"I look different, but I feel more like myself than I ever have in my life!"

The three women, perched on those high stools beloved of talk show directors, smiled radiantly into the television cameras. Dave, the talk show host, and I stood on either side of these makeover contestants as the TV monitor flashed the "before" picture of each "Cinderella," as he had dubbed them. There was a gasp from the studio audience. Yes, once again, the "after" results of my Close-up Makeovers were astonishing.

"I can't believe that you did all this in just one day," Dave said, "and without the aid of a plastic surgeon!"

The studio audience laughed politely.

Dave coaxed some personal "my husband *loves* the way I look" stories from the makeover winners—then there were fast-paced questions from the studio audience. But just for a moment, my mind wandered and I thought: *This is the fifth time I've appeared on Dave's show, the umpteenth makeover contest I've orchestrated, and yesterday was a twelve-hour day at the*

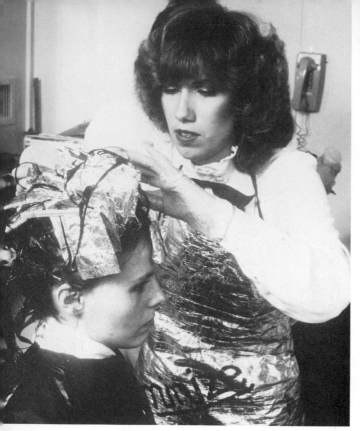 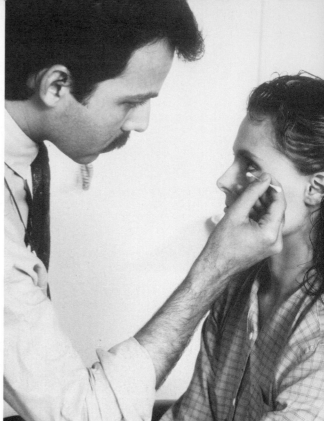

salon. Tomorrow, I jump on a jet for Chicago and do this all over again. And you know what? I love it!

No matter how many times I see my Makeover magic at work, it's always exciting, always fun, and always gives me a feeling of being *so lucky*. What a privilege to be the catalyst who can bring so much happiness and positive change into another woman's life.

How did it all start? From an early age, I've been fascinated with the power of image. In fact, my own life has been a series of self-makeovers, starting when I first dimly realized that, unlike me, my older sister had eyelashes out to *here*, and naturally curly hair.

I was stage-struck, too, and at age ten wrote and produced several plays, held casting calls for the neighborhood children, painted scenery and sold tickets. Years of ballet classes and school musical productions followed, then on to costume design and drama at UCLA. I won several national costume design contests, and was one of five lucky students chosen to study with Edith Head. A twelve-time Oscar winner, one of the all-time greats in the world of design, she was a genius at creating cos-

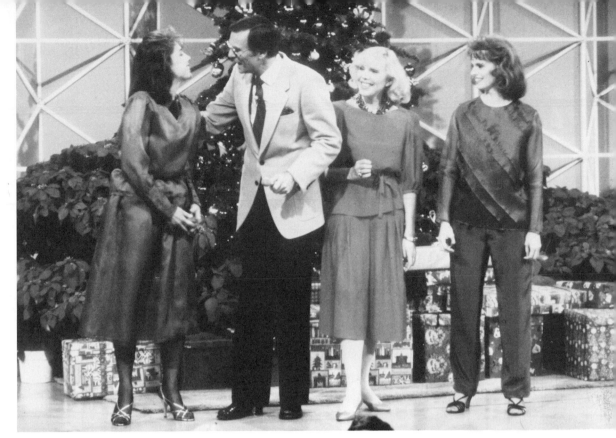

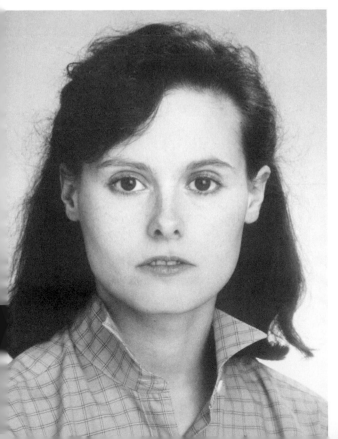

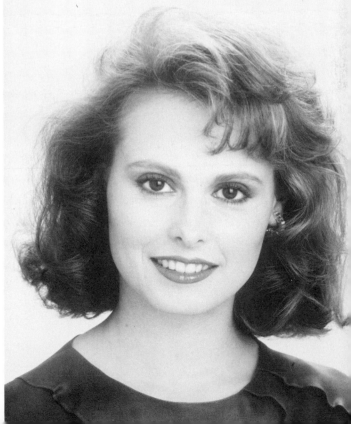

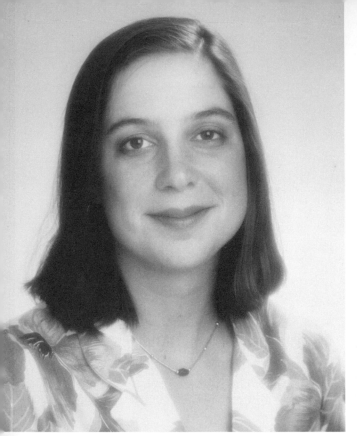 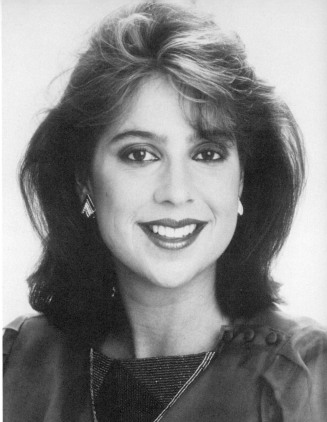

tumes that expressed, rather than overwhelmed, the characters in a movie plot. From her, I learned the countless details that add up to a precise visual message.

And I learned something else, too. My fabulous fantasy designs, so praised by the university's fashion department, were roundly criticized by Head.

"No! No! No!" she fairly shouted, waving her famous trademark glasses. "The look," she said, "has to express a *real* person, with an inner life and character." She replaced the heavy black-rimmed, tinted glasses with a flourish. "And remember, Gloria, always design for the *close-ups*. That's where all the drama—all the important action—takes place."

Her inspiration meant a great deal, not only to me personally, but to so many other women *I* taught. In my real life, and reel life, her invaluable and life-shaping advice has made the most beautiful sense.

My own career followed a dual path, as I raced back and forth from Southern California's sportswear industry where I worked as a model, sketch artist and designer, to acting classes, auditions and eventually to regular appearances in television commercials and as hostess of my own TV talk show. But the two parallel paths came happily together one day when a friend of mine, a much-in-demand lecturer on fashion and beauty, became ill. I was asked to be her last-minute replacement and, without any conscious idea of what I would say or do, I dressed to the nines, drove madly to Beverly Hills, sailed out onto the stage and started talking to 500 women about the image philosophy I had developed, step by step, in my dual career. As I spoke, suddenly it was all there—the program of personal development that combined the practical, down-to-earth fashion concepts of California's sportswear designers with the intensely individual, creative image language of the film industry. They loved it. And they loved it because it was real and I was saying what they wanted and needed to hear.

We are all meant to live fully, beautifully, triumphantly. And one of the first steps in the realization of our true selves is to express our best through our outer images.

"But isn't this accent on the exterior person shallow? Vain? Self-centered?"

I've heard this question in a hundred guises over the years. I can answer firmly, without hesitation: "Changing your looks for the better can change your life." I can be so positive because as I continued to develop and refine my image program, as I taught classes at UCLA, seminars at the University of California at Berkeley, developed my own Image Dynamics courses, and spoke to groups and conventions throughout the country, I have seen countless real-life examples to prove this is true.

When my book *Winning the Age Game* was published, letters from all over the world again reaffirmed my Close-up Image program. I have continued to be fascinated by the impact of image on personality, and when I researched a later book *New Beginnings: Cosmetic Surgery for Men and Women,* I traveled extensively in Europe and the United States talking to cosmetic surgeons about the positive personality impact of an improved outer image. More than ever, I realized the overwhelming importance of the face as a communication tool—with the self and with others. This, then, became the foundation of my makeover system. The realiza-

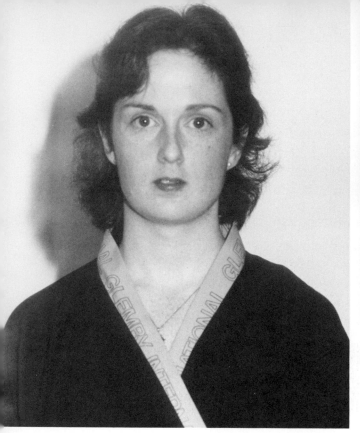 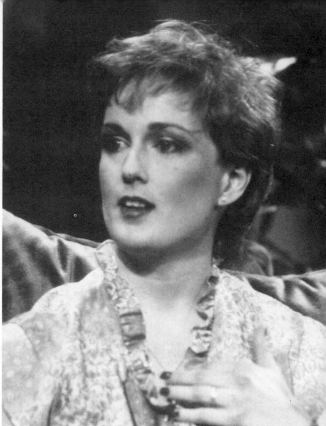

"I never dreamed I could look and feel so terrific."

tion that your face—your close-up—*is saying what you want it to say about you,* can release personal power and bring about a resurgence of self-confidence.

Five years ago, the Clairol Corporation heard of my books and image programs. They, too, have done in-depth research on the impact of image and wanted to bring these facts to the public in a consumer information program. With them, I developed the national television makeover concept that you've probably seen on either local or network television.

These programs, along with my lectures and seminars, have taken me over a quarter of a million miles, to every metropolitan area of the United States. In each appearance, I've attempted to share *everything* I know about makeovers with my audiences. But the question always comes up, from the audience or a TV telephone call-in, "How can *I* have a Gloria Heidi Close-up Makeover?"

This has always been such a difficult question for me to answer. Last year in Detroit, where I chose the makeover subjects from the studio audience, two harried ladies rushed in just after the choices had been made. "Are we too late?" one gasped, out of breath. "We saw you last year," said the other, "and we got up at 4:30 this morning and drove 100 miles as fast as we could to get here."

Of course they were disappointed. So was I. I'm always disappointed that I can't choose everyone in the audience for a Close-up Makeover. Sometimes my television makeovers are part of a city-wide contest. This spring in San Diego, a very young secretary, almost in tears (and on camera, too!), said, "I've entered this contest four times, and today I took off from work on the chance that I might be chosen. Please choose *me!* I want to be a winner."

These emotional dialogues occur whenever I appear in a city to perform Close-up Makeover magic. How can I share my Close-up Makeover program with all of you? This book is the obvious answer. *Every woman reading it can be a makeover winner.* You can learn and perfect the simple, unique program that I've discovered in my life-long beauty odyssey.

When is the best time to start your Close-up Makeover? Without hesitation—and I really can't say this too often—don't wait. Start *today*—which brings me to the very first life-changing attitude in my program.

Take a close-up look at your immediate goals. Rearrange your priorities today. Your Close-up Makeover is going to give you the power to accomplish many positive goals, some you haven't yet dared to dream of. So don't wait to start your makeover until after you've lost weight, changed jobs, gotten the children through high school, college, graduate school! Don't wait until you've accomplished other important goals. Start your makeover *now*. The positive changes in your looks—really so simple to accomplish—will motivate you to move ahead and make other, more important changes in your life.

I could almost recommend a makeover as the first-step in a foolproof diet plan, judging from the number of letters I've gotten from former makeover winners telling me of the pounds they were inspired to lose *after* a successful Close-up Makeover.

Other makeover graduates have changed jobs, gotten promotions, or improved their personal relationships—in other words, put some *zing* back into their love life. I have a zillion stories from very self-satisfied makeover wives: "My husband said, 'I can't wait to get this beautiful blonde into bed.'" Another husband told his wife: "I feel like King Solomon with his own Sheba."

One woman with whom I worked was a very studious-looking, successful CPA in partnership with her accountant husband. Lydia had obviously read all those dress-for-success books, and her appearance sent a loud and clear no-nonsense message. After her Close-up Makeover, her drab hair was shining, subtle makeup gave her a healthy glow, and a colorful blouse added a touch of warmth and vitality to her banker's gray tailored suit. Small changes really, and thoroughly in keeping with her business image, but they brought about big changes on the marital front. As we stood together just out of camera range, waiting for the floor director's cue to show the TV audience her makeover results, Lydia, looking absolutely glowing, handed me a crumpled piece of paper. "Gloria, this was on my pillow this morning," she stage-whispered. "My husband has *never* done anything like this before." The creased note, in his masculine scrawl, said, I LOVE YOU, PRINCESS.

Sometimes, a woman's motivation to make positive changes in her life comes in an unexpected guise. Ann was one of my makeovers whose entire image was a cry for help. I don't mean that she was grotesque, or even terribly unattractive. It's just that she suffered from what I call the LBW syndrome. The Little Brown Wren is the image that tells everyone that the woman within has become totally submerged.

It reveals a life style where self-sacrifice has become a literal description of the inner being. We all know women like this—they have become living sacrifices to their family's needs. Everything in her life is "for the children," and her relationship to her husband has deteriorated to that of a self-effacing household servant.

Ann was a prototype of the Little Brown Wren. Even her taupe blouse and gray polyester pantsuit carried out the theme. After she was announced as a contest winner, I called her house to set up her salon schedule for the following day. Her husband answered the phone and grumped, "Lady, I admire your courage in trying to do something about Ann," he laughed sarcastically, "but it'll take you three years, not three days, to improve her."

Grrrr. No wonder Ann looked the way she did. Her three teenage children proved to be similar ego-killing elements in Ann's life.

Nevertheless, Ann's Cinderella adventure was launched the next day. First, I had the salon change her drab, graying hair to a lustrous, rich brown. Her formerly sallow complexion now had an ivory cast, and subtle blushers made her look full of energy and vitality. But this newly dynamic image wasn't just a simple physical change. Her sparkling eyes telegraphed the inner magic that was taking place. Ann's "after" dress was available in three flattering shades, so I asked her to choose the one she liked the best. What did she want? Red!

As she sailed out of the salon, Ann looked like a new woman. Her body language proclaimed a new-found confidence and self-approval. Still, as the staff and I waved goodbye and sent her on her way home to *that* family, I admit, I worried about her reception. Would their practiced, ego-deflating tactics ruin the beautiful beginning Ann had made? Or would the family suddenly change? Would the children become supportive? Would the boorish husband suddenly realize what a treasure he had? I could hardly wait until the next day at the TV studio to find out.

Ann arrived in the dressing room on time and in good spirits. I directed some quick touch-ups, and she again had that Close-up look that was so flattering, so energizing.

"Well, how did your family like the results of your beauty day?" I'm afraid that my voice had the artificial joviality that doctors reserve for the very ill. Frankly, I shuddered to hear what comments could have come from that negative bunch—afraid to hear that their strong reaction would mean that Ann's makeover would be one of the rare ones that didn't "take," that the entire experience would become a minor one-day miracle, a fond and wistful memory for her declining years.

"How did my family like it?" she said, repeating my question as she looked in the mirror. "Ernie," she called to my makeup artist, "what was the shade of eye shadow you used on my uppper lids? Oh, yes, April Violet." She added a note to her detailed makeup diagram.

"Yes," I said, "but what happened when you—" But Ann interrupted, still involved with her makeup plan. "You know, Ernie, I think this smoky gray pencil will be best for evening, don't you?"

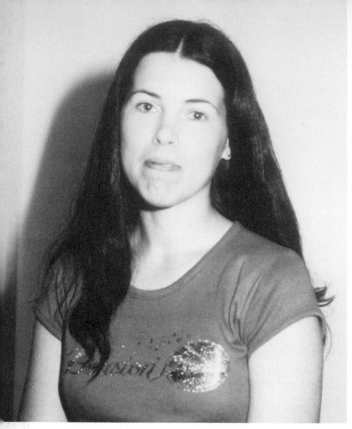
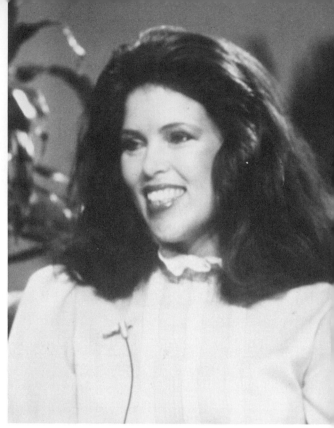

"This is a part of my life I'll always treasure."

By this time, I was periodically plucking at her sleeve. "Ann. *Tell* me."

Finally she said, "No. They didn't like it much. In fact, they didn't like it at all." To my surprise, a satisfied grin lit up her face. "But who cares? I love it. I love the way I feel and I love the way I look. And I'm going to keep looking and feeling this way." Her voice had a new quality, a perceptible edge. "I figure that it's my turn."

I never heard the subsequent chapters in Ann's story, but there was something about the set of her jaw. I just know that, finally, the real Ann had emerged, to live and experience her own life. She would no longer be satisfied to hover around the edges, living her life through others.

These are just a few of the true makeover stories I will share with you throughout my book, stories that prove time and time again, that learning to express your truest, most attractive image, works a kind of magic to bring about life-enriching results. The next Cinderella story could be yours. So don't wait—start your Close-up Makeover program today.

Two

The Success Secret of Your Close-up Makeover

Why do some makeovers "take"? Why do some image changes last and last—and become a life-changing tool? And why do others, equally effective on the surface, fail to become part of a woman's personality? The answer lies in the two essential ingredients of my Close-up Makeover that you'll learn in this chapter. They will guarantee that your Close-up Makeover will be a success. But it's interesting that just as some cooks inadvertently leave out one or two ingredients when sharing a recipe, so all of the makeover experts leave out the two ingredients that are absolutely necessary for the success of your Close-up Makeover.

You may be thinking: "But this is a beauty book. Let's get on with it. Where are the diagrams? The color charts? The lip lines?" They're on their way, in good time. But without developing the two success secrets that I will describe to you now, the technical directions of a makeover are useless to you. That's why it's so important that you read (and reread) this chapter. Open up to the attitudes I'll be showing you now and your makeover results are guaranteed.

How can I be so sure that my Close-up Makeover program will work for you? Why, with so much information available, will my plan bring results where others have failed, or at the very least, left you stuck some-where in a beauty limbo between "before" and "after"? The secrets that I will share with you now are an entirely different approach to the chal-lenge of changing your image for the very best. They give you the miss-ing elements which insure positive, exciting beginnings and life-changing, lasting results.

Success Secret Number One: Inner Beauty

Mother was right when she said, "Beauty starts from within." But there's something mother didn't know. The concept of inner beauty means not just thinking good thoughts and being a nice person, which will certainly reflect on your face, but it also means developing your "Beauty Es-sence"—an inner conviction that you *can* be your most attractive, most effective self. This awareness, the very substance of personal attrac-tiveness, frees a woman from lingering doubts and feelings of uncer-tainty about projecting a new beautiful image.

This uncertainty is a common, in fact a very prevalent, feeling. We've all seen it demonstrated at one time or another in our lives. What mother hasn't felt dismayed to see her newly beautiful daughter, at last wearing flattering schoolwear, reject the neat and pretty winner's image because "it isn't me"? And if you've ever participated in a club fashion show, you've seen examples of the ugly duckling who can't wait to tear out of the makeup and costume that have turned her, if only for an afternoon, into a beautiful swan.

Of course, serious problems of self-image are not the realm of this book. What we will be working with are the all-too-common timidities that keep the average woman looking, well, average. And that's all wrong, because no woman is *average*. Each woman has her own beauty. And your Close-up Makeover is designed to release your unique beauty in a way that no other program has before. You do this by developing your per-sonal *Beauty Essence*. This means learning to respect your desire to be-come your most attractive, most effective self. It means gaining the confidence to put your best face forward and the courage to project the positive image that is the true you. After all, what's the point of learning how to look fabulous if you don't have the confidence to carry it off? Throughout your Close-up Makeover program, I'll be giving you a series of inspiring, motivational exercises that I call Beauty Essence Workouts. These workouts are designed to develop your inner beauty right along with the outer beauty changes that make your Close-up Makeover a unique experience in self-discovery. You will find that the exercises below will help you start to develop those beautiful attitudes that will make your inner beauty unfold.

GIVE YOURSELF PERMISSION

The first step in any makeover is to give yourself permission to change. Sounds silly, doesn't it? After all, you are reading this book because you want to change your looks. Right? Don't be too sure. You can't be different—beautiful, fabulous—unless you give yourself permission to be so. Can you do that? Dr. Eric Berne, author of that perennial best seller, *Games People Play,* says, "The most important element in mental health is to give yourself permission to love, to enjoy, to get the most out of life." And my friend Maggie Morrison, editor of *Family Circle's Great Ideas* magazine, told me, "In interviews with hundreds of women on various subjects, I find that women have difficulty in being good to themselves."

This book is all about being good to yourself. And the first step is to give yourself the gift of beauty. Can you take it? Let's see.

CHRISTMAS IN JULY

This little exercise was developed during a summer seminar that I taught with fascinating, and occasionally hilarious, results. At the beginning of the ten-day session, I asked the workshop participants to think about a gift for themselves. Each student was to set a price level—it could be anything from a dollar to five dollars to a hundred dollars, or whatever her budget would allow, and she was to buy herself a gift within the next three days. It was to be totally self-indulgent. It would not be something that she could use at work. It would not be something that would benefit her family. It would not be something that would add to the value of her home. It was to be a gift for herself alone.

Well, the results were fascinating. One woman had set an eight-dollar limit for herself. She went out and bought an eight-dollar Christian Dior lipstick. She was absolutely thrilled with this purchase because even though she had a good job and her husband was a well-established businessman, she had never allowed herself to purchase anything but dime-store cosmetics. Now, this isn't an argument for buying the most expensive cosmetics. The lesson she learned was that for no valid economic reason she had been denying herself something that gave her great pleasure. She also became aware that she had not been treating herself as a very special woman, one who deserved to have what she could afford. She discovered that she was not a dime-store lipstick lady, but a Christian Dior beauty.

Another woman in the class had great difficulty in buying a gift for herself. Each day I asked her, "Marian, what gift have you bought today?" And she would have some excuse—she didn't know what to buy, she hadn't had time, she couldn't find a store that appealed to her. It was obvious from her outer appearance that Marian had difficulty in seeing herself as a woman worthy of beauty, worthy of expressing her very best image. By day eight it began to be a high point of the class: "Marian, have you bought your gift yet?" We would all wait eagerly to hear what creative excuse Marian had developed that day. She was not able to buy herself anything that was totally self-indulgent. Finally, on day ten when I asked Marian "Have you bought yourself a gift today?" she stood up, took a deep breath, and explained defiantly to the class, "Yes, I finally called the contractor today and I'm having a fence built around my house." There was rather nervous laughter as everyone but Marian immediately realized what a revealing statement this was. She was not only unable to take a tiny step toward self-indulgence, but she was also building a fence to make sure that no other new ideas threatened the status quo. You will not be surprised to hear that Marian's makeover was not successful. She balked every step of the way. Each physical change that was an obvious improvement, that created a beautiful image for her, was emotionally unacceptable.

Not so with Rhonda. She was open and enthusiastic to every step in her makeover plan. And when we asked her on day three what gift she had given herself, she explained, "I went out today and bought a sports car." Well, so much for Rhonda—she didn't need help to be self-indulgent! But, after all, it was a purchase she could afford, she wanted it, so she went out and bought it. Not a bad philosophy.

Now, I want *you* to give yourself a gift! Whether it's a lipstick or a limo (fifty dollars to rent one for an afternoon of shopping!) or a satin jogging shirt marked No Sweat or a dozen daffodils—give a gift, in the next three days, to Wonderful You! Then see what happens. I guarantee you'll find out something interesting about yourself.

F-U-N! CAN YOU TAKE IT?

The next aspect of inner beauty that I'm going to discuss is one that creates in every woman a magnetism, a warmth, and an ineffable charm that can make her irresistible. I'm talking about the ability to have fun. And it's not as common a quality as you may imagine. In fact, this child-like, carefree, open attitude is one of the first casualties of an overburdened sense of duty and responsibility. Fun or play is an important part of your life at any age. Psychoanalyst Irwin Rosen, Ph.D., director of the Menninger Foundation's Adult Out-Patient Department in Topeka, Kansas, says: "The development of a healthy capacity to play is as important an area for the promotion of self-growth as are work and education." So I urge you to approach your Close-up Makeover with a sense of fun, with a sense of play. Recognize that the inner beauty that you will be developing and releasing throughout your Close-up Makeover will occur, not with any real effort on your part, but rather as the result of an open attitude, an attitude that gives you permission to play and to enjoy. Your Close-up Makeover is going to be fun. Can you take it? Test your pleasure quotient on the questionnaire below to increase your appetite for fun.

MEASURING YOUR P.Q.

1 The man in your life gives you a gorgeous, expensive, handmade sweater that is immensely flattering to you.
- You put it away in a drawer. Somehow there never seems to be an occasion that warrants your wearing it. _____
- You wear the sweater with a good suit or with jeans or whenever you choose to feel pampered and special. _____

2 You plan to take a night-school course just to add some interest and stimulation to your life. There are two courses open to you. One is "Foolproof Guide to Preparing Your Own Income Tax" and the other is "Handwriting Analysis and Your Astrological Sign." Which class will you choose to take? _____

3 How good are you at pampering yourself? Have you ever treated yourself to:

A manicure   _____
A pedicure   _____
A facial   _____
A massage   _____
Your favorite perfume _____
A dozen daffodils   _____

4 Do you have some special pamperers in your home? (A cozy corner with pillows in your favorite colors; a small table for your tea; a good reading light, a bath tray filled with luxurious bath oil, a bath pillow, a loofah sponge.) Yes _____ No _____

5 Do you have a room or an area in the home that is *yours*—not the family room, not a corner of the kitchen, but a place that is truly yours? Yes _____ No _____

6 "I don't have a room, corner, etc., nor do I have bath-time luxuries because my husband/children would object, get into them, etc." Yes _____ No _____

7 If you live alone, analyze your environment. Have you made an effort to make your surroundings attractive, comfortable, a frame for Wonderful You? Does your environment reflect your personality? Or are you "just camping," marking time? Yes _____ No _____

8 Do you have a rigid schedule for recreation—tennis every Saturday, dinner with your family or in-laws every Friday night? Yes _____ No _____

9 What is your idea of an ideal evening? _____

_____

How long since you've spent an evening like this? _____

10 Name some event you attended "just for fun" in the last month (Ah, ah—family commitments don't count.) _____

11 You are shopping with your daughter. You find two handbags—one inexpensive and serviceable, and one elegant bag on sale, a real value but more than you'd planned to spend. Your daughter finds *another* decorated T-shirt (her tenth?). Who ends up with what? (Be honest now!)

_____

12 Your husband, your children, your mother, and you have all made conflicting plans. Whose plans are likely to prevail? _____

13 Do you have at least one friend that you can confide in, have fun with, really be yourself with? Yes _____ No _____

Do I really have to tell you the correct answers to these questions? *You know what they should be.* In every case the correct answer means that you should be exhibiting the same generous and affectionate concern for yourself that you would extend to your best friend. Am I saying neglect your family? Not at all. In fact, if you really love them you'll reverse those doormat attitudes that create selfish, inconsiderate children and boorish husbands. And if you live alone, remember the famous old proverb: "Living well is the best revenge."

Success Secret Number Two: Objectivision

Another means of self-discovery lies in developing a more objective awareness of your physical image. All great beauties and those women we all know who look so great, who are at home with their own personal style, have developed this skill. It's the secret weapon of beauty professionals and professional beauties. I call this skill Objectivision, and now you can have it too.

Developing the ability to analyze your looks objectively will take you a giant step toward completing your own Close-up Makeover with thrilling results. Not only is it helpful in improving your personal beauty routine, but Objectivision also helps you to evaluate the beauty services that you purchase from others. When the hairstylist tells you that the style he has just completed, the one that makes you look as if you and Toto have just stepped out of a tornado and into the Land of Oz, makes you look *simply* marvelous, your Objectivision will give you the confidence of your own taste. You will arrive at an opinion based on the firm foundation of self-knowledge. You will be able to say to Mr. Mario pleasantly but firmly, "No, I don't look terrific and I want you to alter the style here— and here."

The four following mirror exercises are the basis of your Objectivision skill. They will help you raise your Eye-Q and develop your ability to see your face, your individual features, and your hair with the Objectivision of professionals.

Here are the props you will need: one large standing mirror—a dressing table mirror, a bathroom mirror, etc.; one hand mirror large enough to give a good reflection of your total facial area; several sheets of plain white typing paper; an old lipstick that is disposable.

EYE-Q EXERCISE #1. HOW TO RECOGNIZE YOUR UNIQUE FACIAL SHAPE

Pull your hair away from your face with a headband. Stand approximately two feet away, or an arm's length from the large mirror. Look directly into the mirror and close one eye. Looking now at the outline of your face, take the lipstick and, holding it at arm's length, start at your hairline and draw with the lipstick on the mirror image of your hairline. Following the outline of your face, come down around past the eyes to the cheekbones; the lipstick is following the mirror image of your jawline, up to the other cheekbone, then back to your hairline again. Now, look at the lipstick outline that you have drawn on the mirror. If you have done this exercise correctly, you will find that you have drawn a diagram approximately two inches wide by three inches long (depending on the shape of your face) that exactly repeats the outline of your facial shape. Take one of the plain sheets of typing paper and place it over the lipstick outline on the mirror. With your finger, press down on the lipstick outline to transfer it to the typing paper. You now have, in Eye-Q Exercise #1, an accurate depiction of the shape of your face. Voilà!

We will be using this diagram throughout your Close-up Makeover to help you choose the most flattering hairstyle, to guide you in all makeup application, and finally to give you clues on what necklines and jewelry will be most flattering to you.

If the outline seems less like the diagram of a perfectly normal attractive woman (that's you) and more like a squiggly portrait of a pregnant amoeba, let me remind you to *keep one eye closed* as you draw your outline, and to concentrate on *drawing the lipstick line at the very edge of your facial reflection.* Keep trying. I promise, you'll get the hang of it. And what a relief to know finally the true shape of that face you live in. P.S.: The lipstick drawings on your mirror will come off easily with a couple of squirts of any standard glass cleaner.

EYE-Q EXERCISE #2. HOW TO ANALYZE YOUR INDIVIDUAL FEATURES

This mirror exercise will teach you how to see the true size and shape of your eyes, mouth and nose. You will also be able to see clearly which side of your face is the most attractive. Then you can use the art of makeup to bring the less attractive side up to standard, as you will learn in your step-by-step makeover.

Again, stand in front of the large mirror (headband still holding hair back), facing straight into it. Now, hold the hand mirror about twelve inches from your cheek. With your *face* still pointed directly at the large mirror, turn your eyes and angle the hand mirror until you can see the large mirror reflection in the hand mirror.

Steady now. You may not thank me at first for revealing this before-now-hidden portrait of yourself. You will find that the image you see in the hand mirror is very different from the reflection you are used to seeing in your favorite mirror, or store window reflections. When I tell you that the hand-mirror image is the face you show the world, you may wish to end it all immediately. But wait. Trust me. The outside world sees basically the same kind of pleasant not-too-bad reflection that you're used to observing, but with every feature and contour simply reversed. There's no need to get a complicated analysis of this phenomenon; the point is that suddenly your eye has been jolted into looking at your face and features in a new way. You'll be using Eye-Q Exercise #2 in some detailed and specific ways as you go through your Close-up Makeover. But for now, do a quick self-analysis to become accustomed to looking at That Face in an objective and professional way.

Analyze the total impact of your facial contours. Is the left side obviously much fuller than the right side? Is your chin very pointed, rounded, or a bit smaller than it should be? Is your nose placed straight on your face or angled a bit to the left or right side? Look at your eyes. Which eye is larger? Yes, everyone will find that one eye is larger. Check out your eyebrows. Is one eyebrow placed higher than the other?

Can you see how all these observations will help you throughout your Close-up Makeover? They will be your guide to choosing the most flattering hairstyle, in applying blusher to widen or narrow your face, to shaping your eyebrows, to widening your forehead, to using highlight and shadow to accent or minimize various facial contours. You will even know whether to try specialized hair coloring techniques to visually alter and enhance your facial shape.

EYE-Q EXERCISE #3. HOW TO ANALYZE THE SIZE AND SHAPE OF YOUR EYES AND BROWS

Hold the hand mirror in your left hand about seven or eight inches from your face. Take the lipstick and, with one eye closed as you did in Eye-Q Exercise #1, use the lipstick to draw an outline around both eyes and eyebrows in the shape of a long rectangle. Take another sheet of typing paper, place it over the lipstick outline that you have drawn, and press down to transfer the outline to the typing paper. You should have a rectangular shape approximately one inch wide and three inches long. With scissors, cut the paper out of the center of the rectangle and shape the sheet of paper so it fits over the hand mirror. You should now have what I call an "isolation mask." When the paper is placed over your hand mirror, the rectangular hole will allow you to look at your eyes, *and only your eyes,* thus isolating them from the rest of your features. You will find that you can look at your eyes and eyebrows in a totally new, analytical and objective way.

Using your isolation mask, take a moment now to really look at your eyes. Do they appear to be large or small? Do they turn up at the corners or do they droop down? Are the eyelids heavy, fleshy, or do they seem to disappear as you look straight ahead into the mirror? Now look at your eyebrows. Do they seem to be too heavy, too dark? Do they dominate the small picture that's revealed to you in the isolation mask? Are they messy? Do they seem too light, too sparse to create a meaningful line?

Can you see how, on Day 5, Eye-Q Exercise #3 is going to help you to create the most beautiful, most flattering eye makeup you've ever worn?

EYE-Q EXERCISE #4. HOW TO ANALYZE THE SHAPE AND PROPORTION OF YOUR LIPS

Follow the directions for creating an isolation mask as given above, but this time use your lipstick to draw a rectangular line around the reflection of your mouth. Place this isolation mask over the hand mirror to get a true picture of your mouth. Look now at the shape of your lips. Are they full or a bit thinner than you wish? Is the outline pouty and rounded, or more angular? Is the upper lip too full to be in pleasing proportion to the lower? Or is the lower lip full, the upper lip too narrow? Realize that you are seeing this feature more clearly than you ever have. And *seeing* is the first step toward enhancing any feature.

Congratulations! You have just taken the first step in creating your own Close-up Makeover. You are becoming an expert on *you,* and it is this personal expertise that will make it possible, literally, to see your smiling face in a stunning "after" picture.

Three

Spotlight the True You

The heart of your Close-up Makeover is *you.* And learning to see your unique physical image through Objectivision is the first step in expressing the true you. But now I am going to take you a step further on your way to beauty awareness.

Most of the makeovers you see are failures—that is, they don't last—because they do not fit into a woman's life style, and most important, *they do not express her beauty temperament.*

Trying to express your inner personality through an inharmonious or unrealistic image is the reason for most makeover failures. Think about it. Haven't you had beauty experiences that didn't "fit," and therefore didn't last and didn't make any contribution to your quest for positive self-expression? The secret ingredient of your Close-up Makeover is *you,* and the ability to match the outer image to the inner woman is the reason my program has been so well received—not only by audiences, but also by the makeover models themselves. That is the challenge I have faced in translating a face-to-face personalized encounter into a formula that you can wrap up, take home, and act upon all by yourself.

As I work on every woman, I ask myself, what are the clues, the symbols, the messages that are the keys to her unique beauty self? What direction should her makeover take? Much of the information is obvious—home life, work schedule, etc. But many of the beauty decisions come from intuition. I've thought about this process and found that the image clues usually point to one of six beauty temperaments—what I call Close-up Portraits.

Discover Your True Close-up Portrait

The Close-up Portraits are a series of descriptive pictures much like astrological profiles. You will find, immediately, that your Close-up Portrait will give you an insight into your own style—an insight that will transfer, visually, to an unmistakable sense of self.

Is there only one Close-up Portrait for you? As you read each portrait description, you will respond to one with a sense of recognition, possibly with wry amusement. "That's me, all right. . . ." But you will probably find that you are attracted to more than one Close-up. Pay attention to your inner feelings, because this is a signal that another side of your personality yearns for expression. Good! Go with it. One of the joys of your Close-up Makeover is in realizing the infinite possibilities that are You.

If you've always been a no-nonsense, casual beauty but find yourself attracted to the idea of being an alluring, irresistible beauty, well, then, now is the time to try! Let the seductive, super-feminine image in this portrait help you express a new aspect of You.

A more down-to-earth reason for casting yourself in several portraits is that the pattern of our lives is not always the same. In my own life, I use several Close-up approaches to my image. When I'm writing, with only a few necessary errands to take me into the outside world, I wear my casual image. A special evening calls for an alluring image. My conferences with TV people require a contemporary look.

The portrait gallery also simplifies your makeover because every single element in your Close-up Makeover is related to a specific Close-up

Portrait. You'll see how this technique will solve many of the beauty and image problems that have kept you from expressing your self effectively. The challenge of matching beauty themes is why makeup, hair styling, wardrobe—all the many elements that go into building an image—can seem so confusing. Well, that uncertainty is over for *you*.

You'll immediately see how hair color, hair style, foundation, lip color, eye makeup, clothes—all these little details—follow the theme of a particular portrait. The result is that professional, pulled-together, total look that translates your beauty temperament into image reality.

Now, step into my Close-up Portrait Gallery and choose one, or several, portraits through which you can express your own beauty temperament.

The Truly Natural Beauty

If you ask the Truly Natural Beauty to describe her philosophy, she will look at you with grave, clear eyes and say quietly, "Well, I just like to be me." The simplicity of this answer and the unaffected image that goes along with it belies the depth of the TNB's beauty temperament.

Natural Beauties, through the simplicity of their lives and of their images, are expressing an almost mystical devotion to nature. An idealist and a dreamer, her sense of self is not strongly centered. She strives to express a harmony with natural things, and her image embodies a process rather than a result. In other words, the wool skirt that you admire is more than an item of clothing. The Truly Natural Beauty may well have raised the sheep, carded the wool, spun the yarn, and woven the cloth. The end result is more than an attractive skirt—it's the expression of a life style.

YOUR BEAUTY PROFILE

Whether quiet and self-possessed or fun-loving and vivacious, one senses a detachment as the essence of your image. You are striving to step away from the turbulent, kinetic present and into a less complex past. You are the true romantic in our portrait gallery. You may live on the twenty-seventh floor of a high-rise in Manhattan and be a top-flight computer programmer. Still, as a Natural Beauty, you will spend weekends baking bread and will plan ahead in November to plant bulbs that will bloom and herald the spring.

When it comes to self-care, the romanticism of the past moves you to make elderberry flower rinses for your long hair, or your own potpourri. Perhaps for a really big evening you may twist your long uncoiffed hair into braids studded with cinnamon sticks for a natural fragrance. We can all learn from the serene life style of the Truly Natural Beauty. Still, if you are a TNB, throughout your Close-up Makeover I will gently urge you to put one foot into the present. The reality of your life is that, more than likely, you are not living in an idealistic commune in the foothills of Santa Barbara. Much of your life is spent in the aggressive, industrial, twentieth-century world—smoggy, fluorescent and neon-lit, noisy and frantic. Your gentle image makes you appear too vulnerable. Remember, a hard-edged image can be an asset, both visually and emotionally, that helps you fit into the real world that, after all, you do occupy.

Finally, a little less of the Puritan would be a very attractive addition to your image. Being open to some of the good things that are part of the contemporary world is not a betrayal of your devotion to the natural essence of life. Recognize too that nature is not always simple and un-adorned. Examine a snowflake or an orchid and you will realize that nature can be very exotic indeed. And nature uses artifice as a beautiful woman uses makeup—a spider web beaded with dew becomes a jeweled wonder that even Tiffany would envy. In other words, if nature doesn't disdain artifice, why should you?

MY ADVICE

If you are a Truly Natural Beauty, you can look glowingly healthy while your otherworldly qualities surround you with an intriguing aura of romanticism. Delicate coloring, clear candid eyes, and softly flowing, uncontrived hair are part of your image at its best. At your worst, as a TNB, you can look pale, tired, even ill—just the opposite of the ideal you are striving to express. Your beauty concept is often too fragile to stand up to the glaring lights of the twentieth-century world. Also, unadorned perfect skin, shiny hair and bright eyes must be the result of true health. Don't just give lip service to the ideal of health. You must *live* it.

Your look can be boring and countrified if you allow it to just happen. Designers like Laura Ashley and Perry Ellis express TNBs at their best. Start a collection of ads and editorial fashion pictures of these designers as an inspiration and guide. Remember, the biggest psychological problem with TNBs is that they are very passive about their image. "Be natural" so often translates to "do nothing." "My brows? Oh, no, I never shape them. I just want to be the real me." But where is the line between laziness and idealism? Dear TNBs, if you want to express nature at its very best, you must take an active stance. Don't be timid about it. Being a Truly Natural Beauty is not a passive, do-nothing statement. It's a positive, active commitment to an ideal.

The Casual Beauty

The Casual Beauty says, "I know I've gone beyond the age and naiveté of looking totally natural, but that image still attracts me. I love the uncontrived, this-is-me message it projects. And frankly, I'm really not that devoted to makeup. I just want to use a couple of makeup techniques, one or two products, brush my hair on the run, and whoosh, I'm out the door."

YOUR BEAUTY PROFILE

Dynamic, active, you're the spark-plug for committees, the save-the-day young executive in office crises, the totally committed parent. Energy, enthusiasm and a whirlwind of activities characterize your life style. (And more than likely you play a terrific game of tennis.) This sense of self can be a plus in your Close-up Makeover—you will probably race confidently through in nine days instead of ten. And the time-saving Close-up plan tailored for you will help you do it. A negative factor is that somewhere along the line, a disdain for self-nurturing has developed, probably because you never have enough time to do all the interesting and demanding things on your schedule. Come on! Pamper yourself a bit. You've earned it. And you'll return to your activities refreshed and renewed. Finally, the very self-awareness that creates your obvious self-confidence can make you inflexible, closed to new ideas. "It's not me," "I *never* wear mascara," "This is the shade of lipstick I *always* wear"—these are familiar lines I hear from Casual Beauties. Now is the time, with your Close-up Makeover, to open up new facets of your personality.

MY ADVICE

If you are the Casual Beauty, at your best you can look classic—a sort of grown-up All-American Girl with polished hair, squeaky-clean skin and sparkling eyes. At your worst, you can look messy and unfinished. And, unless your basic materials are quite good (clear skin, good eyes, straight, nice teeth) this Close-up Portrait offers very few places to camouflage unattractive features. To carry out this Close-up, you must be meticulous about maintenance (haircuts *exactly* every six weeks; eyebrows tweezed and shaped every morning). The few cosmetics you do use must be applied precisely, neatly, not sloppily. Clean, polished maintenance is your theme. Perfect it, and you'll be rewarded with a better than natural look—where the True You comes through.

The Contemporary Beauty

The Contemporary Beauty says, "I think big, I dream big. And I know how to make those dreams come true. I want it all. Not a job but a career.

Not a ho-hum home life but a rewarding emotional life. I don't need to be convinced of the impact of image. My experience in the world of work has taught me the power of packaging. I just want to know how to present the package that will get me what I want."

YOUR BEAUTY PROFILE

Strong-willed, determined, organized, you carrythe glow of success. Wherever you are on your career ladder—everyone knows you're a winner. Even if you haven't put a foot on that ladder yet, you know, though no one else does, that you're going to climb to the top.

The organizing skills that bring you success at work carry over into your beauty life. And you will have great success with your makeover program because you understand the importance of setting a goal, following through with action, and setting time and space parameters. A negative factor here is that you naturally tend to be conservative rather than impulsive. (Your stock portfolio sports names like IBM and AT&T—no Antarctic gold-mining stocks for you.) But your logical and conservative approach to your goals can translate into a predictable, boring, drone-like image that is not the winning ticket. Remember, real leadership involves daring, risk, and yes, shaking up the troops once in a while to remind them that they may not know you as well as they think they do. It's very important to rethink your success image if you are still following that Dress for Success nonsense we were treated to in the '70s. Today's successful woman knows that she doesn't have to dress as a mini-man to accomplish her goals. As a Contemporary Beauty you're comfortable with the idea that you are a successful, accomplished *woman*.

If you are the Contemporary Beauty, at your best your image is elegant, understated, a sleek, pulled-together self-confident look that says you understand power and you express that power in your clothes, in your accessories, in yourself.

Your look depends on meticulous grooming and attention to detail. And your time is valuable, so you organize your beauty life as you organize your career. The Contemporary Beauty is very comfortable about going to experts. Your executive talents have trained you to *listen* and use the advice they give you.

MY ADVICE

As a Contemporary Beauty, you use every talent, every advantage, every skill to be successful. Just remember, Contemporary Beauties can be too successful at forging a formidable image. The Close-up Portrait that works so effectively in your business life does not translate well to your personal life, where the payoffs come in emotional experience rather than goals accomplished. To be truly successful, your life must have balance. And I urge you to study carefully the Close-up Portraits of the Natural Beauty or the Alluring Beauty. These roles are in strong contrast to the hard-driving, ambitious, carefully calculated portrait that expresses your beauty temperament. Think about buying *un*tailored lounging pajamas or something slinky and luxurious. Think of changing to a tousled, free hairstyle after-hours. Not just for someone else, but for yourself.

We've all heard a lot about networking. And what do successful, accomplished Contemporary Beauties talk about when they get together over a business lunch? "My god, where are all the good men?" The Alluring Beauty knows. Think about it.

The Designing Beauty

The Designing Beauty says: "One of my greatest joys is putting my artistic talents to work to create my very own look. I recognize that fashion in its truest form is an important decorative art. And as surely as a ballet dancer interprets the work of the composer and the choreographer, I feel that I'm an artist for expressing all of fashion's art forms. I know I have a very sensitive visual sense. I mean, I know when a hem is one-half inch too long, or when my eyebrows are a touch too bold. I love colors, textures, patterns, and I think my taste is highly developed. I started to say I work at my image, but that's not true—it's not work. One of my greatest pleasures is to read each fashion magazine and see what's new. I adore cosmetics, too. And I keep my things in a lacquered antique box. I can't understand women who complain about the time they have to spend doing their hair and makeup. These beauty rituals are one of the most pleasurable parts of my day."

YOUR BEAUTY PROFILE

Whatever the details of your life style—working woman, wife, mother— an important part of your life is devoted to personal expression. You, the Designing Beauty, have made a career of beauty. You use your creativity to make yourself a beautiful object. Nothing is too much trouble for the Designing Beauty to finish a look, to create a fashion and beauty master- piece. You order one perfect eye shadow color from an obscure theatrical makeup company, brushes from a Japanese artist's shop, and are first in line for the makeup try-ons at your local department store. Using a mixture of creativity, ingenuity, and sound fashion knowledge, you draw upon hairstyling, makeup, and clothes as the raw materials for compos- ing a walking work of art. You have a strong sense of self, but it's more cerebral than sensual. While the Alluring Beauty is always aware of the man in her life and dresses for him, and the Contemporary Beauty is aware of her career, you, the Designing Beauty, are aware of *yourself*.

Designing Beauties are often misunderstood. Acquaintances may be envious and call you vain. Or that girlfriend who is a Casual Beauty may complain: "Why do you want to put all that goo on your face? We're just going to play tennis. Throw on a bandanna like I did and let's go!" Vanity isn't your game though the sparks of admiration that surround you are very pleasant indeed.

Your friends may not understand your beauty temperament, but I do. You are as idealistic as the Truly Natural Beauty, an artist devoted to a beauty ideal.

MY ADVICE

If you are the Designing Beauty, you combine all the best that is contemporary fashion and move in an aura of confidence based on knowledge. You know that soon everyone will want to look the way you look today. Designing Beauties seldom if ever strive to be pretty, but rather arresting, stunning, fascinating. If you have the confidence of fashion savvy, this is a wonderful image for a woman who doesn't have the greatest face in the world. Fashion enables the Designing Beauty to turn plain into pizazz!

To be truly successful, you must pay your dues. The confidence to carry out your dramatic, fashionable, individualistic image comes from knowledge that you must work to acquire. If you want to win the fashion game, you must do your homework. Also, fashion means a total look, from the top of your head to the tip of your toes. But some women are Casual Beauties from the neck up, Designing Beauties from neck to hem, and Alluring Beauties from hem to shoe. Don't mix your metaphors. Your Close-up Makeover will show you how to express your Designing Beauty image most effectively. If the image of the Designing Beauty is one that you have always secretly admired but felt somehow inadequate to express, the steps in the Close-up Makeover will teach you how to do it.

The Alluring Beauty

Ask the Alluring Beauty the essence of her image and she probably won't answer you in so many words. Rather, she'll give you a potent, sidelong glance that seems to say, "I am Woman, and I revel in this glorious role."

YOUR BEAUTY PROFILE

Your hair, your perfume, your clothes, your manner—like the elusive rustling of a red taffeta petticoat—all whisper "vive la difference." The ad line that says, "Part of the art of being a woman is knowing when not to be too much of a lady," could well have been written by you. Provocative, self-aware, sensual, the true Alluring Beauty also knows the importance of subtlety.

The essence of your allure starts with your attitude. And after all, isn't that the first erogenous zone? Still, you're a real, live woman. And you don't spend your time lounging on a chaise, nibbling bonbons. No, you work. And you work out (but a bottle of Chanel No. 5 is the first item that goes into your exercise bag). One might find you joining a climbing tour of Mt. Everest—all those gorgeous men!—but you'll get up a teensy bit early each morning to apply mascara to fluttering lashes. And the fur hat you've chosen just happens to frame your face in a devastatingly alluring manner. Can you help it if every man within yodeling distance is fantasizing about you? A more down-to-earth scenario will find you choosing a look for work or play, but whatever the scene, you will never wear anything that doesn't flatter you and call attention to your femininity. Even if you're happily, monogamously committed, as the Alluring Beauty you always have a swarm of admiring bees circling around the honey.

More sensual than cerebral, at least where your beauty temperament is concerned, you have an intuitive awareness of what is sexy. You know something that your more earnest sisters do not: vanity is sexy. A good healthy dose of self-esteem is terribly attractive to men. It creates an aura of conquest that they find irresistible. And like the Truly Natural Beauty, not only the result but the process of creating your beauty essence is very pleasurable to you. You're devoted to your own healthy body. After all, those hormones have to be pampered! And when it comes to time, you take languorous enjoyment in performing beauty rituals. Joyful, fun-loving, pleasure-seeking, you will thoroughly enjoy all the steps in your Close-up Makeover.

MY ADVICE

As an Alluring Beauty, you have probably spent a lifetime perfecting the art of personal adornment. Ever since age four when you broke into

Mommie's makeup kit and played with all those fascinating grown-up lady's toys, you have made a detailed study of which colors are most flattering, which fashions reveal your figure to its best advantage. Sexy, yes. Stupid, no. In fact, your brains are the most exciting thing about you. Brains and beauty are the ultimate combination for any man with an IQ over 80, and you've used your good brain in a self-analysis that started back in your girlhood.

Subtlety and restraint are the two key words of advice that I would pass along to you, Alluring Beauty. The lure, the game, the chase can become so engrossing that you lose a sense of proportion. Throughout your Close-up Makeover I will be showing you how to avoid the cliches that can make the Alluring Beauty's image a shout for attention rather than an unspoken, self-aware female essence. Appropriateness can be another problem for Alluring Beauties. Volumes have been written about sex and the working woman's image, so I won't belabor the point except to remind you that dressing to bag the Big Game in the working world can be costly in terms of your own accomplishment.

The Ageless Beauty

"I am a rebel," the Ageless Beauty will tell you, a warm smile softening the confident edge in her voice. "And rather than deciding to grow old gracefully, I have decided to grow *up* and be myself." Yes, the Ageless Beauty is an elegant revolutionary, confidently showing the world by her inspiring example that the mature woman of today is unique.

YOUR BEAUTY PROFILE

You will find Ageless Beauties running in the Boston Marathon, chairing a meeting at the UN, writing a steamy first novel that cracks the best-seller list. "It's my turn" is your motto, and you live, finally, to express all aspects of your personality. Now, in your prime-time, you know that agelessness is maturity *without limitations.* You move in an aura of emotional abundance because you recognize that nurturing yourself does not rob the important others in your life of your time, your attention or your love.

Your approach to your enduring beauty reflects your life style and you have no patience with beauty advice designed to squeeze you into the outdated safe little image that much of society still sets aside for the mature woman.

MY ADVICE

Becoming the Ageless Beauty means letting go of old limiting concepts and opening up to exciting new ones. Safe, conservative attitudes are self-defeating and will lock you into a matronly image.

As you progress through the steps of your makeover, Ageless Beauties, I urge you to take cues from several other portraits (after all, you're older, wiser—you've learned that your personality is multifaceted). Pay special attention to the Designing Beauty's portrait. Fashion is the mature woman's best friend. Always remember, image cliches out of the past can make the mature woman look much older than she is—older than she *feels.* But right-now, up-to-the-minute fashion makes you look and feel ageless.

Still, you must make one tiny concession to those candles on your birthday cake. You must become zealous about your health because that is the very foundation of *all* beauty. Your grown-up body cannot build firm tissue, sparkling eyes, and ageless energy on pancakes, coffee or the latest lose-ten-pounds-in-five-days fad diet. So make self-maintenance your avocation. Recognize that it's not a dilettante's choice but a hard reality. Energy, vitality, and robust health are the essense of your profile.

The formula for your successful makeover is this: courage plus knowledge equals confidence. As *Harper's Bazaar* says, "Some of us are reluctant to let go of our old familiar selves, as outdated or inappropriate as they might be, because any change—even one for the better—involves risk." Yes, and risk takes courage. But look, if that risk is based on knowledge (and that's what your Close-up Makeover will give you), what have you got to lose? Only that uninteresting, limiting image that has slowly but surely undermined your confidence, your sense of self. And what will you gain? *You!*

The next step is to decide on your time schedule. You can script your makeover in ten consecutive days—a great way to keep the momentum going—or you may stretch it out to five or ten weeks, which is better for groups because the commitment to a class keeps you motivated. And if this all sounds too structured for your taste, that's all right too. The important thing is to make some specific commitment to take action. Remember, you've already taken the first step—you're reading this book. Directing your makeover means actively taking charge of your image— and that's a way of taking charge of your life. Let's go!

If you would like to organize a Close-up Makeover Workshop, write to me for information.

Gloria Heidi's Image Dynamics
P.O. Box 255–827
Sacramento, CA 95865

Four

DAY ONE

Colorful You

What is there about a woman's hair that makes it the most influential feature in her image? "Starting at the top" says it all. When people look at you, it's your hair they notice first. And your hair *color* attracts more attention than anything else you wear, say, or do. Think about it. Hair color gives you an identity, an image. Specific hair colors surround a woman with a mystique of beauty that, without any conscious effort on her part, send a myriad of powerful and positive beauty messages about her.

But more important than what other people think is the fact that beautiful hair color makes a woman *feel* terrific about herself. I've seen this magic happen every time I direct a makeover.

Does She or Doesn't She? Should You?

It's no secret that I'm sold on hair coloring. I can't help it. I've seen the magical effects that hair coloring has on a woman's image and on her

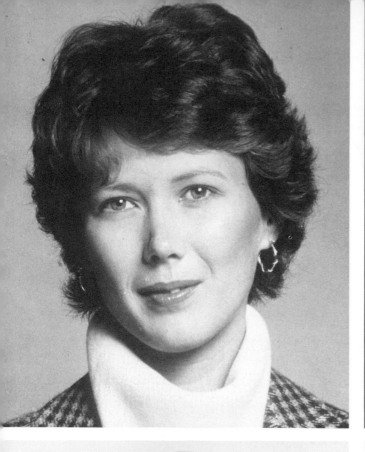
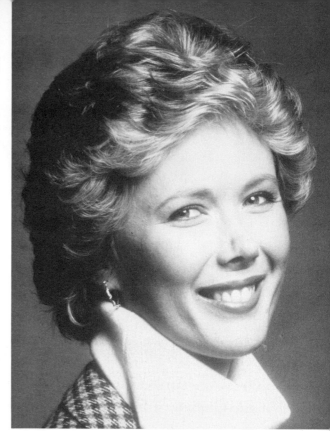
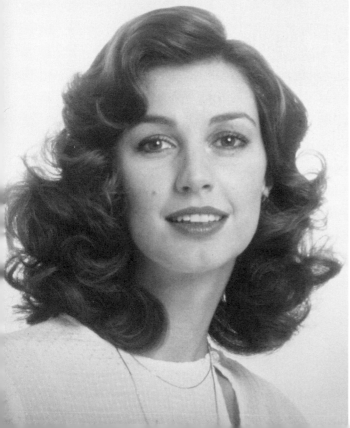
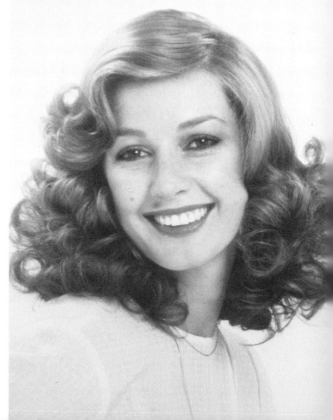

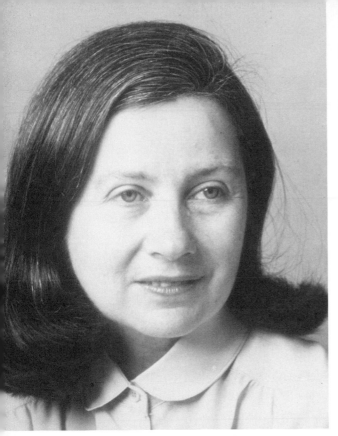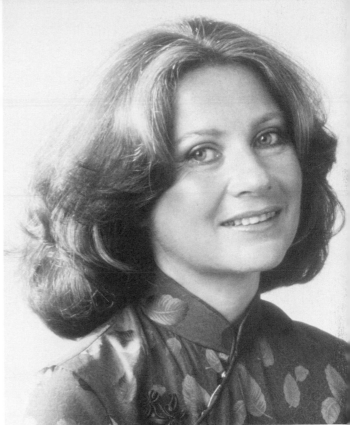

Like contemporary makeup, today's hair coloring gives you a subtle and natural look.

psyche time and time again. The bottom line is this: hair coloring is the fastest, easiest, most inexpensive way to make an immediate positive change in your appearance. Diets take months. Clothes cost hundreds of dollars. And plastic surgery—well, that takes money and nerve too. But with hair coloring, in less than one hour you can create an immediate, believable, exciting change in the way you look and feel. It's a modern miracle, and it's no wonder that one in three women in the United States uses some form of hair coloring product. Specifically, this is what hair coloring can do for you.

1   Hair coloring enhances your skin tones. It absolutely turns on the lights in your complexion.

2   Enhanced hair coloring sets the theme for your personal color scheme. When hair coloring is right, all other elements in your personal palette come into focus.

3 Hair coloring maximizes the beauty of your hair on every level, including texture. The conditioners in contemporary hair-coloring products will make your hair shiny, silky, and add volume and body as well.

4 Enhancing your hair coloring has a remarkable effect on your sense of self. Perhaps that's not so hard to understand when you realize that hair color is the way we establish our visual image. People say, "She's a blonde," "She's a brunette," "She's a dear little gray-haired lady." When we *choose,* through the use of a hair coloring product, to change from an indeterminant image (dishwater blonde, for example) to a definite one, somehow we are beginning to have a clearer sense of self.

How does hair coloring accomplish all these miracles? The answer lies in the new attitudes about its purpose. Hair coloring used to be surrounded with a veil of secrecy. Disguising the color of the hair was often the main reason for doing it, and early products often brought about a too dramatic or brazen change. Today, the whole purpose behind hair color is to make your hair the best it can naturally be, and new products make it possible to bring out the most subtle, natural and believable color effects—effects that every woman can live with.

Leland Hirsch, new-product consultant for Clairol, says: "Think in terms of *brightening* your hair color to bring out the complete palette of color gradations in it—not to cover up or drastically change it. Anyone, from the palest blonde to the darkest brunette, can go brighter as long as the effect is natural-looking."

Another contemporary approach to hair coloring is that it's like makeup. New products are subtle and so easy to try that hair coloring is no big deal anymore.

Look at your hair right now. Could its color be more flattering to you? I'm not talking about a drastic change—perhaps just a few shades lighter or darker will please you more than anything too dramatic. Contemporary hair coloring gives you lots of choices, but of course that can be a challenge. Finding the right hair color for you can seem to be a pigment of your imagination.

Color Me Fabulous

Here's how to choose the best hair color for you.

1   Think of what color your hair was when you were a child. It's my feeling that this is your most flattering shade, your natural hair color. For example, if you were blonde when you were a child, you can almost be positive that you'll look terrific as a blonde adult. After all, your skin tones are basically the same. Incidentally, if Mommie has saved one of your ringlets, you can check it to see whether your hair was golden blonde or a very pale Nordic blonde and just what shadings it had. One exception to repeating your childhood hair color: if your hair was very dark when you were little, dark when you were a teenager, and now that you're thirty-five your hair is going gray, you should *not* go darker with hair color. Always go lighter as you get older. And whatever your age, be careful of the very dark shades in hair coloring. Lighter and warmer are your best bet.

2   Do you like what the sun does to your hair? Often women who would like to be blonde love those wonderful sunny summer streaks which are so flattering. And brunettes may find that the sun brings rich auburn tones into their hair. So, if you like what the sun does to your hair, you can achieve those same tones through hair coloring.

3   Winter and summer are cool, spring and autumn are warm. Hair coloring, too, breaks down into warm and cool shades. So if your general coloring is warm tones, you want to stay with warm hair coloring, and if you're cool-toned, you want to stay with cool. But when in doubt, go toward the warmer shades. Why? It's a cold world out there. Most of us live in an atmosphere that reflects cool, blue, unflattering tones. Whether it's fluorescent light, sunlight fighting its way through a blanket of smog, or the cold, impersonal light reflected from the concrete skyscrapers of any big city, creating a personal color aura that is warm in tone will be flattering to almost every woman.

4   This brings me to the last and most important guideline in choosing your hair color—all the experts advise that you change your hair just a few shades to start. As expert colorist Louis Licari pointed out in a recent interview, "When you go to the beach and get a little bit of color people say, 'M' god, you look terrific.' Think about it. When you get that lovely flattering tan, your skin doesn't change eight shades. Perhaps just two little nuances of color make you look great. The same subtle color change in your hair will do the same thing, will give you the same dynamite look."

So change your hair just a few shades to start. You can always do more, and you'll be happy with the slight change to start with. You will find that enhancing your hair color makes such a *fabulous* difference in the way you look that, on an emotional level, it's almost more than you can handle if you do too much at first. Here's an interesting phenomenon—family, friends and co-workers almost never pinpoint enhanced hair color as the basis for your new glow. They just say, "You look wonderful!"

Your Close-up Consultation

The first step in the Close-up Makeovers I do for TV is always a color consultation, whether it be with Louis Licari in New York or Bill Palmer in his salon at the Beverly Hills Hotel, or any number of marvelous colorists in between.

Now you can do as the pros do. The very first step is to decide what your goal is. You'll need a hand mirror, a hair brush, a pair of scissors, and a white index card. Brush your hair thoroughly to remove any hair spray and to fluff it out so that the full array of color and texture will catch the light. Now, using your hand mirror, look at yourself in strong daylight. Study your hair and make some decisions.

- "I want to give my natural hair color more depth and richness."
- I want to brighten and lighten my natural hair color a few shades."

- "I want to go really blonde."
- "I want to add some high-lights."
- "I want to add warmth to my hair color."
- "I want to darken my hair"—careful here.
- "Gray hair is making my own hair color look drab. Gray hair is making me feel old. I want to cover the gray."
- "I want to blend in gray streaks with highlights."

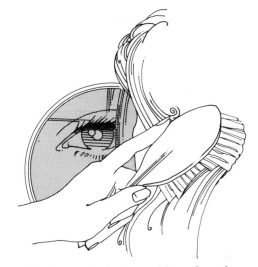

Brush your hair thoroughly and analyze its present color.

Next, use a preview strand to really see your present hair color as the pros do. Snip a small lock of hair (one-quarter-inch wide) close to the scalp from the darkest or grayest part of your hair. Scotch-tape it to-gether at one end, and staple that end to your white index card. *Save this preview lock. You'll be using it on Day 2 to complete your hair coloring.*

Take the strand and really study it in the sunlight and under strong incandescent light. What color undertones can you identify? Are there golden glints? Warm auburn highlights? You may be shocked to see that when you really examine your hair closely it is much drabber than you ever imagined and there may be a lot more gray than you were aware of. And that is the culprit that is making your hair color so uninteresting.

Whatever color effect you want for your hair, there's a hair-coloring product to make it happen. The key is to choose the right product for the result desired. Remember, the foolproof way to successful home hair coloring is to choose a product that will (1) give you the effect you want and (2) fit in with your life style. There's a whole cast of hair coloring products to let you be anything you want to be. When you check out your Close-up Portrait, you'll see that I've made specific product suggestions for each Beauty Temperament.

Having chosen the kind of product and the effect you want to achieve, consult the side panel of each hair coloring to get a preview of how the shade you've chosen will look on your particular hair color. Now, this is important: be aware that the color on the box is not precisely the color you will get. The color on the box is hair coloring applied to pure white hair. The color you will get after using the product will be your unique custom color—a combination of your own hair color plus the color on the box.

Take your preview strand and hold it up to the color selection chart on the package you are interested in. To lighten and brighten your own hair color, choose a shade lighter than your natural color; to darken, choose a shade darker than your natural color; to cover gray without changing your natural color, choose a shade closest to the natural color. It's generally better to select a shade slightly lighter than the natural color because that's more flattering for most people. If your hair has a lot of gray, you may choose to cover it with a shade close to your natural color, but there are many fun and interesting things you can do as I'll explain in the Close-up Portrait for Ageless Beauties.

SPOT ANNOUNCEMENT

IF YOU ARE UNCERTAIN OR NERVOUS ABOUT HOW TO MAKE YOUR COLOR CHOICE, THERE IS A BATTERY OF EXPERTS JUST WAITING TO GIVE YOU ALL THE ADVICE YOU NEED—FREE. CALL CLAIROL'S HAIR COLOR CONSULTANTS ON THE TOLL-FREE HAIR COLOR HOT LINE: (800) 223–5800 (NEW YORK, CALL COLLECT: (212) 664–2990).

There's a good chance that you already color your hair, but as a part of your Close-up Makeover you want to change the present shade. If you've lightened your hair and want to go still lighter, it's a fairly simple matter. Try a little at a time, choosing the next lighter shade in the same family of colors that you've been using. Just be sure to use the same type of hair coloring that you are presently using—do not mix semi-permanent (the kind that blends away in six shampoos) with permanent hair color (the color stays until it grows out).

If you've darkened your hair, it's a little difficult to go lighter. It's easier to lighten the natural pigment of your hair than it is to lighten hair that's been colored. However, there is a product that will remove darker hair coloring. It's called "Metalex" and it's a conditioner as well as a corrective treatment so it will not hurt your hair. In fact, it will make it look and feel better. But for specific directions on how to make a dark-to-lighter color change, I strongly urge you to call the Clairol Hair Color Hot Line for expert direction that will assure the results you want.

If you want to go darker, take it easy. Use a shade *slightly* darker than the one you've been using and gradually ease into a darker tone.

Does Fun Really Have More Blondes, More Brunettes, or More Redheads? Let's Find Out

We've talked about the importance of considering your basic hair color and your skin tone in choosing the hair color shades that will be the most flattering. But now I want to talk about a different aspect of this subject: the mystique of hair color. Is there a blonde, brunette or red-haired personality? I believe there definitely is. And you'll want to check out the blonde, brunette or redhead's mystique before you make a final choice in hair coloring.

Typecasting has always been one of the staple elements in movies and TV. Nowhere is the impact of hair coloring more obvious. There is a cluster of psychological and emotional symbols that surround each of the basic coloring types. Flipping your TV dial from "Dynasty" to "Dallas" to "Hart to Hart" will give you a quick rundown on what I mean. Blonde Krystle (Linda Evans) personifies all the characteristics of the blonde goddess. She's good, she's gorgeous, and she's got her man (this week, anyway!). Alexis (Joan Collins) is the quintessential brunette, mature, knowledgeable—"My dear, one has the feeling she knows *everything*"—and not afraid to use her power. And red-haired Jennifer Hart (Stefanie Powers) is the essence of the impulsive redhead. She races sports cars, jumps out of planes, and solves murders—all with a good-natured flair.

While all this seems part of the realm of fantasy, the powerful impact of hair color in terms of personality expression is something that every woman should be familiar with. The three basic hair-color types influence how people respond to you and can definitely affect how you feel about yourself. As you read my description of the blonde, brunette and redhead mystiques, see which one expresses your beauty essence most clearly.

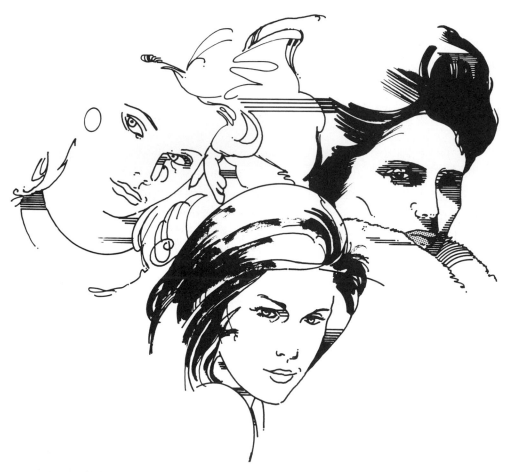

Blonde, brunette, or redhead—the three basic hair colors surround a woman with a definite image.

THE BLONDE MYSTIQUE

Mankind has always been enchanted by blonde womankind. That undeniable mystique has made the fairest of hair a source of excitement and intrigue for centuries.

Why have blondes always been so idealized? Because the majority of all peoples has always been brunette, and therefore blondes have always been visibly different. New York psychologist Dr. Stanley Wicklan says, "The blonde woman is traditionally the idealized woman. She looks different so she is immediately perceived as being more valuable and perfect." In our culture, the blonde personifies the fantasy woman, the one men wish to possess and women aspire to be. The blonde is seen as carefree, fun-loving, and above all, beautiful. Because so many women are blonde as children and their hair then darkens as they grow up, blondeness is associated in our subconscious mind with youth, and darkness with maturity.

UCLA psychiatrist Dr. Roderic Gorney in his book *The Human Agenda* says that the adulation of blondes is associated with our love of sunlight and fear of the night. He states that the blonde image connotes both childhood innocence and sexual abandonment. No wonder gentlemen prefer blondes. But what about blondes themselves? Do these attitudes become self-fulfilling prophecies?

The Blonde Beauty Essence: If other people believe blondes are distinctive, it's not surprising that blondes themselves view their golden locks as more than just a lot of hair. In fact, a recent study revealed that women who lighten their hair actually feel they have a blonde personality. Blondes picture themselves as more outgoing, more feminine and more confident than other women. But there has always been a vulnerability about them, a quality that simply adds to their fascination. I believe this vulnerability is because the woman who *chooses* to become blonde (and after all, most of us do; only a small percent of the population is truly blonde) is well aware that she personifies the ideal woman. Fun-loving, carefree and provocative on the outside, the blonde's beauty essence is still as elusive as quicksilver. She seeks to personify an ideal and so she is always in the process of becoming—a brunette *is*.

Vulnerable or no, today's blonde is different because today's woman has changed. In a recent national survey, it was found that the blonde of the '80s is seen as more than just beautiful, glamorous and sexy. She's also successful, likeable and, new for blondes, intelligent. The expression of this new image is demonstrated by the fact that almost all of the TV anchorwomen, our most visible role models, are blondes. In the past, blondes had more fun; but in the '80s, they have it all—authority, money, and yes, they're still having a terrific time.

If it seems that I'm overselling blondeness, read on. Women with blonde beauty essence know it and revel in their blondeness. But a true brunette wouldn't be blonde on a bet. The vehemence with which they reject blondeness is always surprising to blondes, but it makes perfect sense to strong-willed brunettes.

THE BRUNETTE MYSTIQUE

If Hollywood has crystallized our ideal of blondeness, it has created an indelible portrait of the powerful, magnetic brunette. While blondes are seen as innocent, carefree and childlike, the beauty essence of brunettes is one of maturity, stability and knowledge. That knowledge can be translated into the stereotype of the brainy career woman—think of all those old Joan Crawford/Rosalind Russell boss-lady movies.

Brunettes are also viewed as being very, very sexy, but in an entirely different way from blondes. Even brunette sex symbols have a maturity in their image. In their heyday, Sophia Loren and Elizabeth Taylor were seen as the essence of Woman—a sort of hyped up, super-sexy Mother Nature. Current brunettes—Ali MacGraw or exotic Diana Ross—still embody that double image. While our blonde angel may be naively appealing, the smoldering, mysterious brunette knows all of nature's ageless love secrets. Brunettes are seen as powerful, passionate, fiery, *elemental* women.

Psychiatrist Gorney has this to say about the brunette image. "It encompasses the devoted, stable, mature wife and mother aspects of femininity, but interestingly also includes the darkly mysterious characteristics exemplified by Theda Bara and the Dragon Lady. International spy types or arrogant society ladies and mean stepmothers are usually typed as brunettes. While blondes must be both innocent and sexy, brunettes must be equally contradictory as both motherly and siren-like."

Brunettes are favored in perfume advertising. Nina Blanchard, head of her own top modeling agency, says: "Brunettes somehow embody the seductive image wanted for perfume. Usually in movies the mysterious Other Woman is portrayed as a brunette. She is the dangerous femme fatale . . . she is more mysterious and interesting."

So much for what others think of brunettes. What do brunettes think of themselves?

The Brunette Beauty Essence: There is a basic confidence in brunettes that says, "Yes, I am a woman of *this* world. I know who I am, what I want, and how to get it. I'm confident in my sexuality too. I'm my own ideal and I'm only interested in becoming more definitely myself—a true brunette." The character in *Yentl* who said "women are *born* knowing everything" was definitely describing brunettes.

THE MYSTIQUE OF THE REDHEAD

True red is the most unusual hair coloring shade, and the redhead considers herself a one-of-a-kind woman. "Like orchids, we're unique and rare." Individualistic and unconventional, she says, "I don't have to follow the crowd. I wasn't born to be part of it." Queen Elizabeth I of England embodied the redhead's mystique perfectly. Dynamic, unconventional, with a temper to be reckoned with, she ruled a great kingdom with energy and flair.

Yes, they're fiery and tempestuous, but redheads can also give the image of intriguing contrasts. The classic red-haired look—creamy, fragile pale skin and green eyes in cool contrast to the banked fires of auburn or titian locks—expresses the inner contrasts of the red-haired temperament. In fact, it must have been a redhead who inspired the nursery rhyme "When she was good, she was very, very good, and when she was bad—look out!"

As colorist Licari explains: "I think red is a special color because when it's beautiful, it's so very beautiful. It's the romance color, you know. I always think of the true Raphaelite woman having this beautiful ambery red, gingery hair." He continues, "Red hair is nature's most special, special color for only the most special woman."

I did my own informal survey and asked a variety of men what they think of redheads. Here are some of the adjectives that were used most often: unpredictable, unconventional, impulsive and reckless, tempestuous and fiery. And the flip side—kittenish, foxy, fun-loving. One man summed it up nicely: "Red is a hell of a color. I mean you have to be a pretty sparkly girl to wear it."

The Redhead Beauty Essence: Redheads seem to be passionate about their own hair color. They either love it or hate it. Which is understandable in one way because true "carroty" red hair can be pretty difficult to live with. Also, red is the most elusive color and rapidly fades as time goes by. But there are hundreds of red tonalities in hair-coloring products that will let a true redhead make her hair very glorious indeed.

If your friend Ginger decides to change her current flame-red hair color to a rich, elegant auburn, you can be sure she will decide on the spur of the moment, dash out to an all-night drugstore, buy a new shade of shampoo-in hair color, race through the directions, and have the whole process completed within an hour and a half. And if, when she's towel-drying her hair at one A.M., a friend calls and invites her to fly to Las Vegas for breakfast, your red-haired friend won't think twice. Next stop, Las Vegas.

Yes, the image of redheads is that they are impulsive and fun-loving, and that image, according to one colorist I spoke with, is the reason many outwardly shy, rather introverted women choose to become redheads. They want to express these strong extroverted qualities. If blondes are outgoing and brunettes self-possessed, the image of a redhead is one of a woman who is independent and unconventional. Think of the great movie redheads—Rita Hayworth, whose challenging glance seemed to say "love me if you dare"; Ann-Margret, the sex kitten with claws; Katharine Hepburn, probably the most famous movie redhead, unconventional, feisty, independent and outspoken.

Lacey Ford, of the famous Ford Modeling Agency, told me, "The red-haired models at our agency all seem to know each other very well, to have a sense of camaraderie, to stick together. It's as if they know they are a very special breed, and they understand each other."

Ask a flame-tressed beauty if she would ever consider becoming a blonde or a brunette and the heated answer is, "Never! I'll try any color— as long as it's *red.*"

Hair Color for Close-up Portraits

There is a hair-coloring product to let you be anything you choose to be. And contemporary hair coloring products are as varied as the lifestyles of the women they are created for. So the following are simply suggestions for hair-coloring products that I feel will fit into the lifestyle and temperament of each Close-up Portrait. Use these suggestions as a starting point to investigate your color-full options.

THE TRULY NATURAL BEAUTY

Clairol's Light Effects: a kit that uncovers the natural highlights in your hair. Good news, not just for blondes, but for brownettes, brunettes, redheads. There are four different formulas, each designed for a specific hair color, so choose the one that's made for you and get light effects as natural as the shimmer of lights that the sun puts into your hair.

THE CASUAL BEAUTY

A Frost-N Tip kit will add pizazz to your outdoor look. The sun-kissed results will enhance your breezy image and at the same time fit in with your no-nonsense, time-is-of-the-essence beauty temperament. A Frost-N Tip kit saves time because after the initial frosting it only has to be redone every five to six months. These kits give you many options. You can add a little or a lot of sunshine. Note: not the best choice for brunette

Casual Beauties. If your hair is dark, try the Light Effects kit described in the Truly Natural Beauty's portrait.

CONTEMPORARY BEAUTIES

Clairol's Color Renewal System will enliven and enrich your natural hair color and give it color brilliance that will stand up to those color-draining fluorescent lights.

DESIGNING BEAUTIES

You will find that Clairesse will give you high-fashion dimensional color effects in a whole range of color choices.

ALLURING BEAUTIES

You can choose to become an ultra blonde, an exotic brunette or a dramatic redhead with Miss Clairol. This product will make the most emphatic color statement and offers you the biggest number of options because you can go several shades—lighter, darker, warmer—in any given direction.

AGELESS BEAUTIES

You will find that Clairol's Loving Care covers the gray beautifully and can either turn it into highlights or let it blend in with your natural color, depending on the color choice you make. If your light brown hair is just beginning to gray, you can use a Frost-N Tip kit to add more emphatic dramatic highlights. You'll see that those beginning gray strands will just mingle in with the glamorous new highlights you've added.

Preview of Coming Attractions

Tomorrow, you'll be coloring your hair and preparing for your Close-up hairstyle. The ease, convenience and flexibility of modern hair coloring is indeed wonderful. Still, there are some specific steps that you must take today in order to have the most satisfactory results.

Open the box of hair coloring that you've chosen and get out the directions. Turn to the section entitled "How to Test for Allergies" and carefully follow the simple directions for giving yourself a patch test. Allergies are not common but some people may be sensitive to hair-coloring products, so you must test yourself twenty-four hours before each and every application of hair coloring.

You will also preview your new hair color at the same time. *The only way to know how any hair coloring will look on your hair is to apply the preview test.* Take the small lock of hair that you have stapled to the white index card. Remove it from the card and place it in the color mixture left over from your allergy patch test. Be sure that the tiny strand is completely covered with hair coloring. Carefully follow the directions that accompany your hair-coloring product, especially the instructions about timing. Check the preview strand every few minutes until the right shade is achieved. After following timing directions, if the strand is not the color you want, you may need a different hair-color shade. The point is, *do as salon professionals do.* Check and double-check the amount of time it takes to achieve the hair color that you used on the preview strand.

Once the strand has reached the right shade, let it dry and clip it again to the white index card, noting on the card the exact amount of time you applied the color to the test strand. If you don't like the color, check to see that you've left the hair coloring on long enough. This is a very common error. Still, if it's not what you want, you can switch to another shade. If you do like the results of your preview test, you can go ahead and apply this color to your hair tomorrow, knowing that you will love it.

Day 1— Beauty Essence Workout: How to Rewrite Your Beauty Script

Rewriting your beauty script through positive inner dialogue will program your entire being—physical, mental and emotional—toward the successful completion of your makeover. What is inner dialogue? Dr. Denis Waitley, author of *The Winner's Edge,* and an expert in the psychology of winning, explains it this way. "We're talking to ourselves every moment of our waking lives. It comes automatically. We're seldom even aware that we're doing it. We all have a running commentary going on in our heads on events and our reactions to them." Waitley goes on to explain that the difference between winners and losers, those who achieve their goals and those who fall short, is in the quality of their inner dialogue or, as he calls it, "self-talk." "Winners think constantly in terms of 'I can, I will, I am,' while losers concentrate their waking thoughts on what they should have or would have done or what they can't do."

When your inner dialogue is positive, your mind will go to work to make that scenario come true for you. Mind, body and emotions all respond and will work to carry out the performance of that thought as if it had already been achieved before and is now just being repeated.

That's the principle behind positive inner dialogue, a technique you'll use to rewrite your beauty script. Now let's step beyond the abstract explanation to some action-oriented, specific steps that will start you on your way.

1 Listen! If the idea of self-talk is new to you, begin to listen and pay attention to the running commentary that accompanies every scene in your life. What messages are you giving yourself about your makeover? What messages have you programmed into your being regarding your image? Is your inner dialogue positive—a pep talk from a loving, energetic coach who wants you to win—or is your inner dialogue timid and negative, a cruel critic urging you to maintain the status quo? I repeat: listen! Pay attention! Become familiar with how the plot of your life is being scripted in those 800 words per minute that compose your inner dialogue. *By changing what you are saying to yourself, you can change your life. By changing what you are saying to yourself, you will create that climate of inner beauty upon which the success of your Close-up Makeover is based.*

2 "How can I control my inner dialogue?" Waitley says, "The self-talk of winners is affirmative and directed toward the results they want." Winners coax the mind toward the goal in positive terms and say, "This is the positive way I see myself." Losers, on the other hand, hedge their bets; their inner dialogue is filled with plans to deal with the failure of a project, rationalizations if it doesn't work out, and little sermons designed to dampen enthusiasm for a project so, "if it doesn't work out, I won't feel so disappointed." Even compliments are turned aside and every accomplishment is treated as a fluke. Think about it. Can you accept a compliment? You'd better get used to it because your Close-up Makeover is going to bring you many opportunities to practice this little social ritual.

Try this and listen to your inner dialogue: "You're looking absolutely fabulous! Are you wearing your hair a new way?" Now, how did you respond to that compliment? Practice a negative response. Does that negative attitude feel very natural? Pay attention to that. Practice a flukey response: "The hairdresser had a lucky day. My hair's usually a mess." Now, think of a positive response to that compliment. Does it come easy? This is something you'll want to work on throughout your Close-up Makeover.

Remember, positive inner dialogue is the first step in programming your Close-up Makeover. On the very first day, I want you to be aware of the essence of this beauty program: *what the mind can conceive, the mind can achieve.*

Five

DAY TWO

Glorious Hair: Make It Happen!

Today you will continue the steps that make your hair your most important accessory. You'll start by coloring your hair, carefully following the directions on the particular hair-coloring product you have chosen. Get out the index card with the preview strand clipped to it and the coloring time that you noted yesterday.

When you have finished, shampoo your hair and towel-dry it. Take a moment now to enjoy your enhanced hair color. See how it seems to have turned the lights on in your complexion?

At this point, your first thought will probably be a brand new hairstyle to set off your color-brightened hair. You may want to rush out to the nearest beauty salon or to your favorite Mr. Jacques or Miss Renee and have your hair styled. I can understand how you feel. But right now I'm going to make a surprising suggestion. Wait! So many women are unhappy with their hairstyle because they haven't given it the careful study and analysis that will result in a fabulous finish. Consequently, they have a love/hate relationship with their hairstylists. All over the country I hear complaints about how the hairstylist will not "give me the look I want." Well, stylists are not entirely blameless in this equation, and on

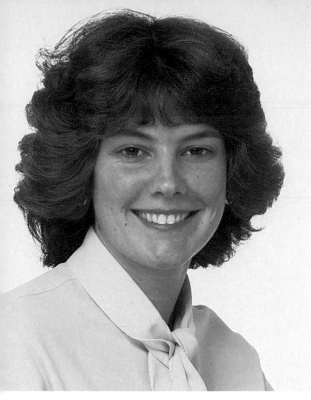
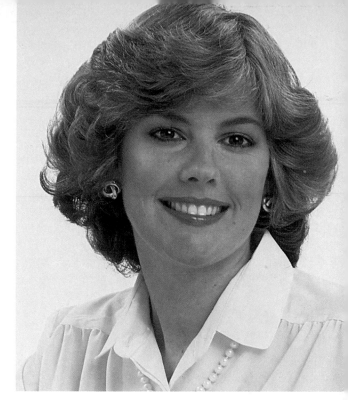

Change your hair color just a few shades to start.

Today's hair color makes your hair the best it can be.

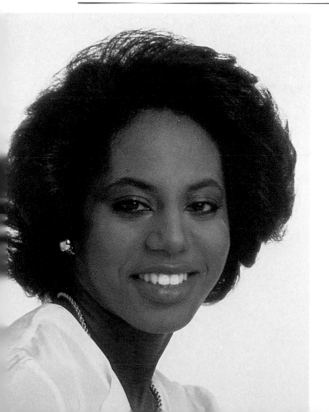
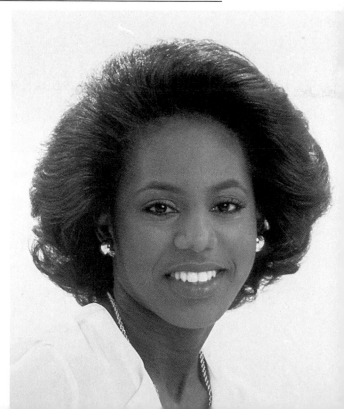

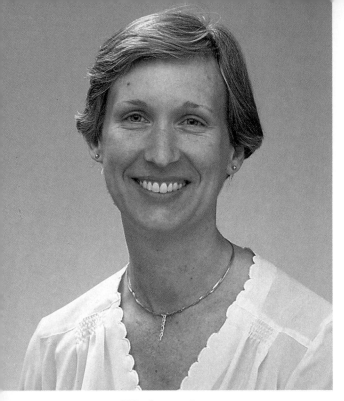
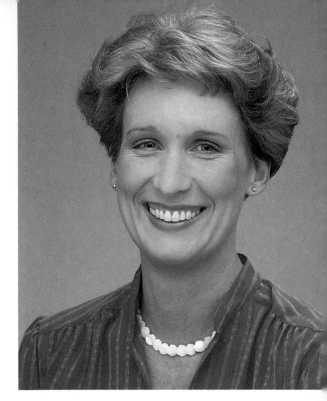

Why be gray?
It's so easy to turn drab, aging hair into a beauty plus.

Turn on the lights in your complexion with a subtle hair-color change.

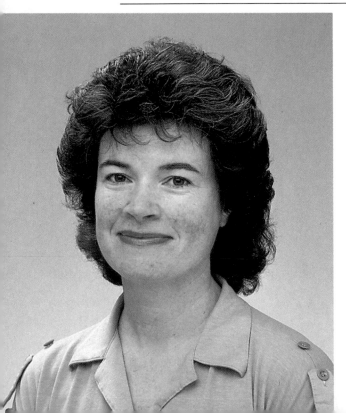
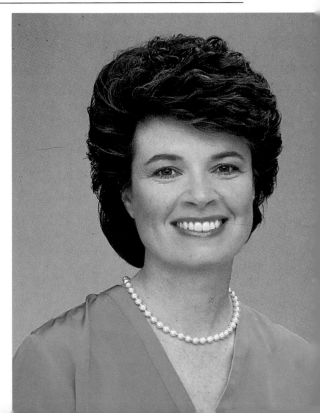

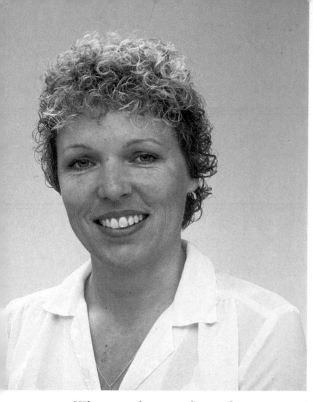

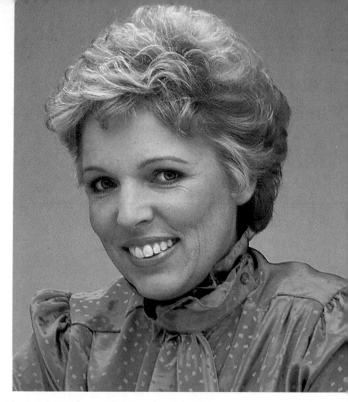

When you choose to change from a vague image (drab brown) to a definite one (blonde), you start to develop a clearer sense of your beauty essence.

A bonus of hair coloring—it adds body and volume to fine hair.

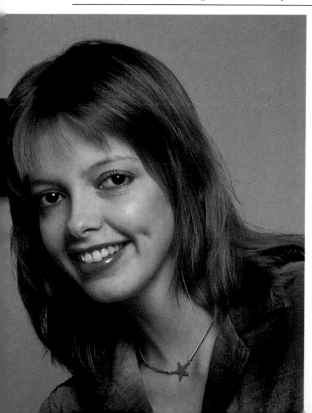

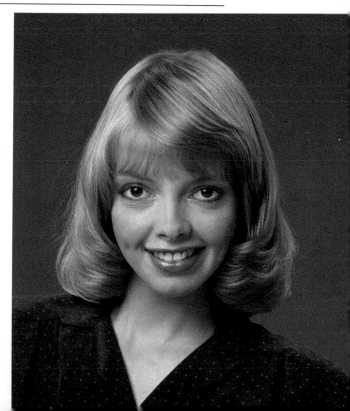

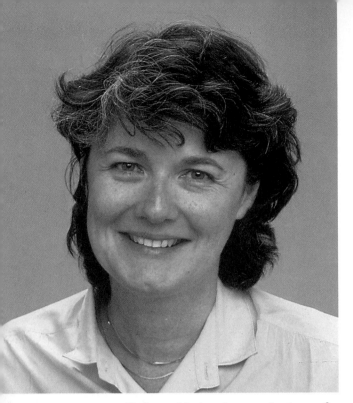

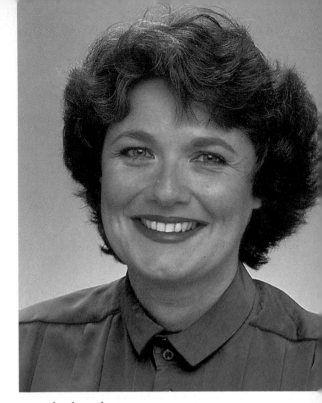

Enhanced hair color sets the theme for your personal color scheme.

Hair color is the fastest, easiest, most inexpensive way to make a beautiful change in your image.

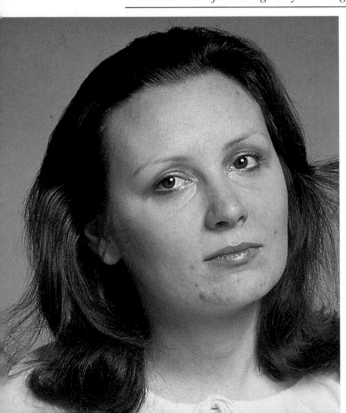

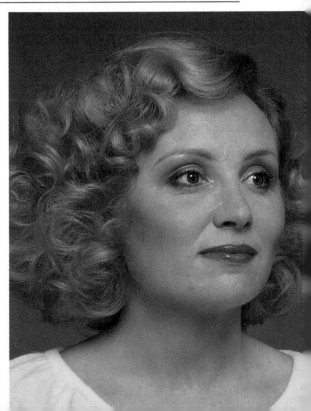

Day 7 we'll be talking about how you can work most effectively with them. But starting today, you're going to do *your* homework. Knowing what you want will take you a long way toward getting it. Today's research will help you determine the hairstyle that will both flatter your physical features and truly express your beauty essence.

Hair coloring will make your hair the best it can be, but it will not change the basic characteristics and that is what we are going to analyze now. Fine, coarse, straight, wavy—your hair type will remain the same with one exception. If you have gray hair, which is often very wiry, you will find that hair coloring has dramatically softened and silkened it.

In choosing how to wear your hair, you must know its characteristics and choose a compatible style. Stylists across the country tell me that the biggest reason for dissatisfaction with hairstyles is that women insist on one that is incompatible with the fabric of their hair. That's why it's so important to be aware of precisely what kind of hair you have. Hair comes in an endless variety of combinations. It can be fine or coarse, dry or oily, the texture may be baby-fine, fine, medium, coarse or even very wiry.

Beautiful Hair — Through Thick or Thin

If your hair is thick, you can easily tell because it *is* a handful. Fine and silky hair, on the other hand, may not *seem* thick because of its baby-fine texture. Here's how to tell. Looking in the mirror, lift your hair up at the roots and look through it along the scalp. You'll know your fine hair is thick if you see that the hairs are close together and that there are lots of them. If your hair is thin, you'll see that the individual hairs are farther apart.

Next, you'll note whether your hair is curly ("It drives me crazy in damp weather"), or straight ("It drives me crazy in damp weather"). Somehow, we're *never* satisfied with what Nature doled out to us. Wavy hair comes in a variety of levels, ranging from the hint of a wave at the temples to a luxuriant wave that starts at the roots and undulates down to the very tip of the hair.

To get an idea of which styles will be right for your hair, think of it as a fabric. The many, many hairs on your head, like the individual fibers in a bolt of material, combine to create certain characteristics. If you sew, you know that style and fabric must be compatible to create a beautiful garment. If you don't sew, just check out the losers on any sale rack and you will often see garments where the fabric and style do not work together. For example, you may see a rumpled, droopy safari jacket sentenced to the mark-down rack because it was produced in a soft, silky fabric that could not hold tailored lines. The same design idea relates to your hair.

If your hair is fine and soft, it is like silk. It will be more difficult to work with because it won't hold the shape of a style. Simple styles, all one length and blunt cut to give the look of thickness, will be flattering to your fine silky hair. A body wave (applied at least ten days after you have used hair coloring) will also add needed body and volume.

If your hair is coarser, it will be similar to cotton fabric, able to hold a tailored shape. Coarse hair is easier to work with, more moldable, and able to hold a curl, so you can probably wear your hair successfully in a number of different styles. If it's very coarse, a layered cut will help reduce the bulk and give your hair a softer, more controlled look.

Straight, limp hair is like chiffon. It has no shape of its own, will not hold a line or a curl, and is a real trial to any woman who has it. A body perm is really the only way you'll get a style to hold. Blunt cuts that are a little shorter in the back with the sides layered for fullness will help this type of hair hold its shape.

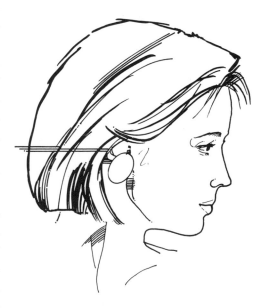

All-one-length, blunt-cut styles are best for fine hair.

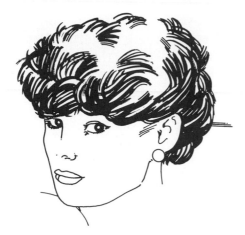

Coarse hair holds the curl and is more versatile.

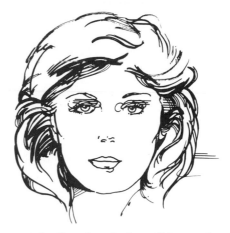

Straight, limp hair looks well in a style that combines blunt cut with layered sides.

Make notes on the information you have gathered and share this with your hairstylist. See? Right away you are going to have a basis for improved communication. One fact will become immediately clear. What you like and what your hair will do may be two entirely different things, so a few compromises may be necessary before you find a hairstyle that really works.

But that is the value of a good professional haircut and styling, one that takes advantage of the natural tendencies of your hair—the natural curls, waves, cowlicks, and straightness. The more you go against the natural tendencies, the harder it will be to maintain your hairstyle.

The Long and the Short of It

As I travel throughout the country working with women in every state, I find that by far the biggest hairstyling mistake women make is to wear their hair too short. So often I must reject a woman as a makeover candidate because her hair is simply too short.

I recently overheard the following conversation while having my own hair done. The women next to me was describing to her stylist the hairstyle she envisioned. "I want it to be waved here on the side and to sweep over my forehead in a sort of waved bang, and be sure it curls around my ears and creates some fullness at the side." The stylist responded to these directions with a series of "Mmmmm's" and "Uh-huh's" and something in their tone made me turn around to take in the situation. "My hair is much too long," the woman was continuing, "and I can't do a thing with it." Well, no wonder the sytlist was so noncommittal. The crop of hair that she expected him to cut and shape into an attractive new style was only one to two inches long all over. Nevertheless, he proceeded to trim a fraction of an inch here and there from this already cropped haircut. He knew, as I did, that if he didn't cut her hair, this woman would go somewhere else and complain that she had paid for a haircut she didn't receive.

What is the reason for this short-cut approach to hair beauty? Many women confuse a hair *cut* with a hair *style,* and when they are bored or unhappy with the look of their hair, they take the fastest way out—cut it to make a change as quickly as possible. If this sounds like your beauty scenario, I urge you to start now to grow that crop of hair so your stylist will really have something to work with. Otherwise it's like trying to make a beautiful dress out of a quarter yard of material.

One final observation on the subject of too-short hair. It's been my observation that women who are overweight often wear their hair much too short in proportion with their larger bodies. This is all wrong. If you are at all overweight, you need enough hair to be in proportion to the size of your face, possibly to camouflage its fullness, and to keep your head in proportion to your not-so-small body. So, if you have a weight problem pay close attention to what I've just said. This is one of the most important bits of image advice I'll give you.

Do I ever see hair that's too long in my travels cross the country? Absolutely, and it's almost always on younger women who are wearing their hair too long to be flattering and too long to make any sort of image statement beyond a rather vague "those years at Peahawkin High were the best years of my life." In fact, *if you're under thirty, you should probably*

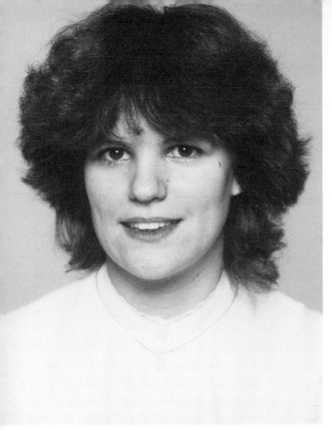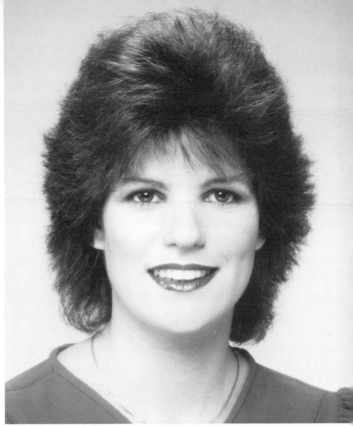

The right hairstyle can dramatically flatter your facial shape.

wear your hair shorter than you are currently wearing it, and if you're over thirty, you probably need to wear it longer.

What Shape Are You In?

Now, let's talk facial shape. As you probably know from all those magazine articles, hairstyles can create fool-the-eye tricks to visually correct less than attractive proportions. A general rule is this: never repeat in your hairstyle a line or shape that you do not want accented. If you have a round face, for example, don't wear a rounded cap of hair or a mop of rounded ringlets. Rather, choose waves instead of curls and a more angular line direction rather than a round one. Use the silhouette and line direction of your hairstyle to bring your facial shape closest to the ideal

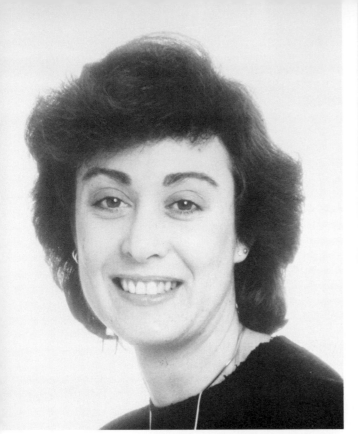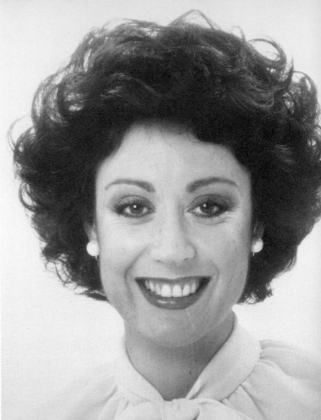

Your Close-up hairstyle can visually lift facial contours.

oval. Of course if you have an oval face, the sky's the limit—you can wear almost any style that will be compatible with your hair's texture.

Now that you finally know the true shape of your face from the Objectivision exercise on page 26, you will be able to choose hairstyling elements knowledgeably.

Brush your hair into its usual style and look into the mirror. How could this style be changed to be more flattering? Move your hair around. Try parting it in different ways. Pile your hair on top. Pull it back. Obviously your hairstylist will know the refinements of these design details—that's one of the skills you're paying for. But this preliminary session will make you more open and receptive to the changes he suggests. Here are some guidelines:

Characteristics of the basic facial shapes showing suggested flattering hairstyles:

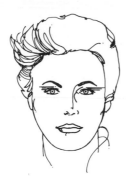

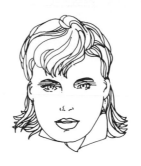

OVAL: *forehead slightly wider than chin*

ROUND: *round hairline, round chin line*

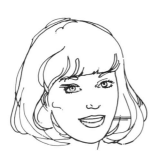

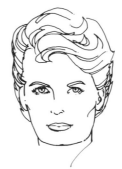

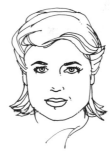

OBLONG: *long and narrow, flat or hollow cheeks*

SQUARE: *square hairline, square chin*

TRIANGLE: *narrow forehead, broad jaw and chin*

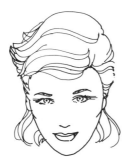

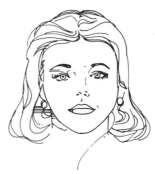

DIAMOND: *wide cheekbones, narrow at forehead and chin*

INVERTED TRIANGLE: *wide forehead, narrow jaw line*

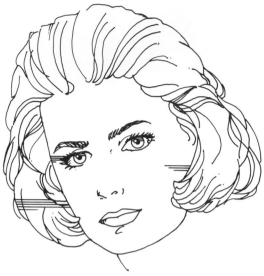

● To make your whole face or just parts of it seem larger, pull hair back. Try pulling your hair back from a too-small jawline or delicate cheekbones. Does your face look larger now?

Pull hair back from delicate cheekbones.

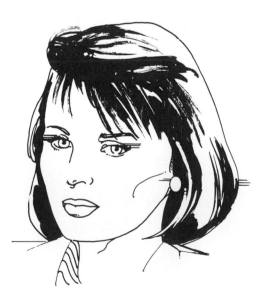

● To make your whole face or part of it seem smaller, draw hair forward. Bangs will minimize a high forehead. Hair brought toward the face at the jaw will minimize full cheeks. Pile your hair on top of your head. See how your face looks longer and thinner, your chin narrower?

Draw hair forward to make an area seem smaller (a square jaw line for example).

● To make a facial area seem wider—at the top, the sides, or the bottom—fluff your hair out and put fullness in that area. Hair that is flatter on top and fluffier at the sides will make your entire face appear to be wider and shorter.

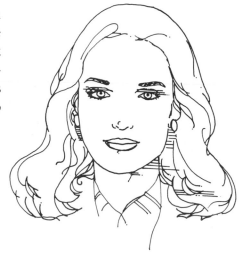

To add width, fluff hair out at sides.

● Look at your profile. Do you have a prominent nose or chin? Counterbalance these two prominent features by adding fullness at the back of the head, toward the crown for prominent noses, opposite the jawline for prominent chins. Prominent noses will also be balanced by curls or full bangs.

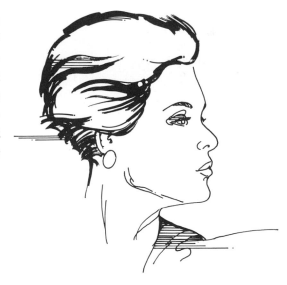

Counterbalance prominent features— noses, chins—by adding fullness at back of head.

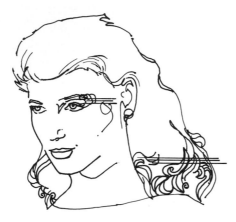

• Receding chins will be bolstered with fullness near the chin line. Avoid curls or bangs at the fore-head.

Bolster receding chins with fullness near jaw line.

• Where you part your hair can also create an illusion of length or width. The closer to the top of your head that a side part is placed, the more visual length it will create. The further toward the side of your head that you part your hair, the wider the visual effect that will be achieved. Center parts are chameleons in this respect. If your face is wide and round, a center part will emphasize the width. If your face is long and narrow, a center part will emphasize the length. Center parts are bad news for almost everyone!

The specifics of this styling job are the responsibility of your hair-stylist, a professional who knows all the many nuances of line, direction, proportion. Your job is simply to become familiar with your face, your features and your hair so that the two of you can confer intelligently and cooperate in arriving at your goal—that perfect, flattering, wearable hairstyle.

Your Close-up Portrait Hairstyle Analysis

TRULY NATURAL BEAUTIES

The musical *Hair* was a hit in the sixties but now, over twenty years later, it's still the theme song of most of the TNBs I see. Hair, hair, and more hair—whether it be beautiful or thin and straggly or bushy and over-whelming—there is just too much unstructured, messy hair in the TNB image. Don't worry, I'm not going to suggest a drastic cut or too much control ("I've gotta be freeee . . ." shouts the TNB). But here are some styling suggestions to bring your look up to date and make your hair look and *be* healthier.

1. Stop parting your hair in the middle and letting it hang! You are stuck in the past if you're *still* wearing this Joan Baez look. I mean, even Joan doesn't wear it that way anymore. A center part is unflattering to almost everyone because it accents every irregularity of your features and will emphasize a long, crooked, or too-large nose. Try a side part . . . and see? Like magic, your face looks better.

2. Let's cut some of that precious hair. Think in terms of shoulder length or, at the most, two inches below the shoulder. That's not so traumatic, is it? Remember, this is not plastic surgery. It'll grow.

3. Even if you want to wear your hair fairly long, do consider having it styled so that it is shorter around your face. You can still look and feel wild and free but with a flattering '80s image.

4. Lots of TNBs have been devoted to the "natural"—that ultra-curly hairstyle made popular in the late '60s and '70s. This look is usually the result of a very tight perm, and that unstructured mop of curls is an appealing image for many TNBs. But check now to see if you have brought it up to date. The look of the '80s is achieved by using *larger* perm rods which will create angelic ringlets rather than tight frizz.

THE CASUAL BEAUTY

"I barely have time to brush my hair, let alone curl it." "When I jog, I *sweat*—and there goes any complicated hairstyle . . ." These are the realities of the CB's beauty life. But too often her solution is a wash-and-wear haircut. And I do mean c-u-t. *Short* is the theme. But you *can* have hair that combines easy maintenance with becomingness. Here's how:

1. Think in terms of a *great* haircut, one that will have a "line" and shape even after you step out of the swimming pool, and will save you hours in daily maintenance. You'll have to book salon appointments every four or five weeks to keep that super cut in the same great shape your body is in!

2. Most wash-and-wear hair is too short and flat at the crown, too long and bulky at the nape of the neck. Reverse this. Hair should be longer at the crown, shorter and shaped at the neckline. Look for styles that have a bit of length (two to three inches) around your face and four inches at the crown of your head. This is a much more flattering and versatile cut, as you will see.

3. Time-saving appliances are your best beauty friends. Hair dryers, curling irons, and especially hot rollers—my candidate for chum #1 on anybody's list. Put two or three hot rollers on your longer crown hair. Do your minimal makeup. Take out rollers and, shazam! You have a flattering hairstyle, not just a practical wash-and-dash cut.

THE CONTEMPORARY BEAUTY

You'll be choosing a hairstyle that works to give your professional image more authority, more clout. Of course, if it flatters you, could it hurt? But the main characteristic of Contemporary Beauties' hairstyle is that it avoids extremes—neither too long, too short, too soft, too severe. The ideal hairstyle is a very conservative version of prevailing fashionable styles, and fashion does play a part in your hairstyling image because it creates an impression of timeliness and social awareness. Still, unless you actively work in the fashion industry, your hair styling choice will be a conservative version of What's New. Here are some specific examples of the kinds of messages your hairstyle can project.

Long Hair. If you like to wear your hair long, look for styles that will create an impression of controlled authority. You might sweep your hair up and out of the way or comb it all back and tie it with a crisp grosgrain ribbon. Both are excellent professional styles that make the most of beautiful longer hair.

Short Hair.   Short, severe no-nonsense hairstyles (those outmoded dress-for-success images) create an overkill effect for the professional woman. True, they do make Contemporary Beauties look hard-working and efficient. But severe hairstyles also create a stern, forbidding and inflexible impression. Soften the severity of short practical hair by adding waves or even curls. Also, remember my advice about avoiding extremes. Hairstyles with a little more length at the crown and especially at the back of the neck will be professional looking but not too severe.

Curly Hair.   Curls are great and they flatter the face. But uncontrolled curls look a little too casual and flamboyant. A good stylist can cut naturally curly hair in a way that will make the most of your curls and yet create a controlled professional and businesslike image.

In fact, if I were to choose one word that characterizes the hairstyle of the Contemporary Beauty it would be controlled. Messy, unkempt hair seems to say "I'm unorganized. I can't be bothered with details." Whether short, long, curly or straight, the Contemporary Beauty's hairstyle will create an impression of controlled femininity and superb grooming.

DESIGNING BEAUTIES

Finding your most flattering, appropriate, expressive hairstyle is the goal of each Close-up Portrait. But Designing Beauties have an additional challenge. Every season designers show new clothes with new themes; every few years they present us with new proportions. The design elements in a hairstyle complete the picture. In essence, hemlines go up and down, so do hairstyles. To complete the picture, your hairstyle must be fashionable too. In fact, the secret of "carrying off" the latest fashion lies in an awareness of the Total Look. All elements of a woman's image—hair, makeup, clothes, accessories—are carefully selected to complete the total design impact.

Aspiring Designing Beauties will find that the fashion magazines spell it out: length, proportion, mood. Read the editorials, study the pictures, absorb the visual details. Is hair full and voluminous, silky and unstructured, short and geometric? DBs are also aware of the tiny little fashion details that can make or break a Look. Just as a hemline that is a half inch too long or short can take the edge off high fashion impact, something as subtle as the diameter of a curl can be important in a hairstyle. The successful Designing Beauty absorbs all of these details.

So, DBs, where your own hairstyle is concerned, you are open to change, either to subtle variations on a flattering theme or perhaps to a big change. Caution: fashions in hairstyles change gradually from one look to another. Be wary of very extreme faddish hairstyles, especially if they require an extreme haircut—it may take years to grow out, long past the time of its fashion impact. So look for fashion, not fad, in choosing your Close-up hairstyle.

Still, if you're going to play the fashion game, it's absolutely essential that your hairstyle change. If you are wearing your hair in exactly the same style it has been for the last five years, you are failing to project the total fashion image. Too many would-be Designing Beauties get failing marks because they don't recognize the *totality* of each design theme. If you're going to play the fashion game, you must play it from head to toe. Your stylist will work with you on this, but you must educate your eyes to accept the visual impact of the New.

ALLURING BEAUTIES

When it comes to sex appeal, hair is the mane event. Sensually, we are often gauged by our hair. In fact, next to your rounded female body, your soft, pretty, touchable hair is your most feminine physical quality. Alluring Beauties know this instinctively. You can't project a feminine image without a feminine hairstyle. Any length can be sexy, and I'll give you the detailed characteristics of alluring hairstyles. But long, loose, luxuriant hair is never read as anything else.

What else is sexy? Tousled ringlets (Bernadette Peters and Goldie Hawn are two examples); tangled manes (Farrah Fawcett, Victoria Principal); long, silky, swinging hair (Christie Brinkley, Crystal Gayle). More: asymmetrical styles where hair is swept behind the ear on one side, tumbled forward toward the face on the other; long hair piled loosely on top of the head giving the impression that a man could remove one strategic hairpin and the glorious mane would come tumbling down; soft waves, baby curls, enticing tendrils at the hairline—all create a touch of Eve in the Alluring Beauty's image.

Health is an essential part of allure. Out-of-condition is unappealing for hair as well as figures. Shiny, bouncy, silky, luxuriant hair is the result of proper hair care. You, the Alluring Beauty, are meticulous about conditioning your hair, having your stylist clip off split ends.

Hair is a universal symbol of sexuality and you must appreciate that the super-sexy hairstyle that proclaims you're a woman may overshadow the fact that you are a lady too. Color-rich, shiny, abundant, gorgeous hair projects a powerful sexual message, and there are many occasions, Alluring Beauties, when you will want to turn down the volume. At work, for example. Study the Close-up Portrait of Contemporary Beauties for some guidelines on how to apply a little restraint, a little control to those passionate locks of yours.

THE AGELESS BEAUTY

The keys to your best hairstyle, Ageless Beauties, will be found in the Close-up Portraits of Designing and Alluring Beauties. Fashionable softness sums it up. Fashion, so that you tell the world you're not living in the past; softness, to proclaim, "I am still an alluring woman."

The hairstyles of so many mature women seem to be reminiscent of some triumph in the past ("Yes, that's a picture of me when I was voted Miss Indiana. I haven't changed much, have I?") But of course you have changed. *Everything's* changed. And thank heaven for that—live in the dynamic present and let your image help you do it. Throughout your Close-up Makeover, you will hear me telling you that fashion is the mature woman's best friend. To determine your best hairstyle, follow the fashion guidelines that Designing Beauties know so well, with these stipulations: never choose the most extreme hairstyle and always choose one with an element of softness.

So many Ageless Beauties have the mistaken idea that facial features that have been slightly blurred by age will be brought back into focus by a super-neat, controlled, rigid hairstyle. Not so. In fact, the sharp outlines of a severe, controlled hairstyle will, by contrast, simply emphasize the softened jawline, that less-than-trim cheek contour. Severe hairstyles are only for those impossibly beautiful actresses and models who would look terrific wearing a motorcycle helmet.

Also take to heart my comments on length. Do not wear your hair too terribly short, especially at the neckline. A severely neat, clipped or even shaved (shudder) hairline is an impossible image for the mature woman, robbing her of a very necessary image element of femininity. If you choose a short hairstyle, look for one where the neckline is taper-cut and left long enough to create a tiny wave or a delicate tendril.

Your professional stylist will be very aware of the camouflage magic that the right hairstyle can perform in counteracting subtle signs of age. Here are a few pointers that the two of you can discuss in order to turn back the clock with your new hairstyle.

● *Double chin and jowls.* Fullness at the crown of the head at about a forty-five-degree angle from the point of the chin will visually counter-balance fullness in the chin and jaw area.

● *Scrawny neck and jowls.* Forget all that limiting advice about "now that you are a certain age, you must wear your hair shorter." True, long flowing locks are not right for you if you are a grown-up lady. But choose a hairstyle that is long enough to cover the sides of your cheeks and shadow your neck to distract from these aging contours.

● *Drooping facial contours.* Hairstyles with an upward direction create visual magic and appear to lift drooping contours almost as much as a mini-facelift. That doesn't mean you should pull your hair straight up on top of your head in an Olive Oyl knot, just make sure that the dominant lines of your hairstyle always have an upward direction. This sounds totally obvious, but look around. See how many mature women are wearing their hair swept back or down rather than up? Even if you wear your hair down at the side, be sure that there is an upward direction created by a lift at the temples, or soft angled bangs, or fullness at the crown of the head. All up-lines in your hairstyle should follow the lines of a forty-five-degree angle that would lead to the crown of your head.

A few Ageless Beauties whose hair has turned gloriously gray or silver do not choose to cover the gray. Though gray hair may be beautiful, it will be an age maker unless you choose a *very* fashionable hairstyle. A super fashionable haircut with lots of verve and pizazz will counteract the "nice lady" image. The move from conservative to chic may be intimidating at first, so ease into it with fashion knowledge and work with your hairstylist over a period of time to achieve a right-now look.

By now you should have a complete picture of the elements necessary to create your perfect hairstyle. Before you go off to the beauty salon to have your hair restyled on Day 7, here are a few assignments to complete over the next five days.

First, start shopping for a hairstylist. If you are presently going to a stylist on a regular basis, now might be a good time to evaluate your relationship. Is Mr. Jacques or Miss Renee taking you for granted? Do you always get the same quick in-and-out, conservative hairstyle, no matter what you ask for? Or is he/she constantly urging you to try a new look? In other words, will your present stylist be open to the new beauty attitudes you are developing? More than likely, your present stylist will be delighted and thrilled to work with you in developing your Close-up hairstyle.

Here are some tips on finding that special salon where your styling will take place.

It goes without saying that if you are already a regular customer in a salon where you feel comfortable, you will probably want to make it the scene of your Close-up hairstyle. Just make sure that Jean-Louis understands you are not coming in for your usual shampoo-and-set; you do not want to walk out looking the same as you do after your regular Tuesday appointment.

But what if you only have a haircut every six months and never in the same place twice? Or you have just moved to a new town, and haven't found a salon? What if you are downright intimidated by beauty salons? How in the world are you going to find the right stylist for you? Believe me, it's not as difficult as you may imagine, and it can even be fun. You know how to shop, don't you? Well, that's what you are going to do: go comparison shopping for a salon and stylist, with "comparison" being the key word.

The first thing to do is compose a preliminary list of stylists who are candidates for your hairstyle. Ask those friends whose hair always looks terrific where they have it done. You can even approach a total stranger and ask her the same question—she is sure to be flattered, and will probably give you a wealth of information about her favorite salon and stylist. Check the better department stores in your area—they almost always have large, well-staffed salons. Look in the Yellow Pages (although this is a last resort—a personal recommendation is better). Ask the cosmetic saleswomen at the department store counters—they are beauty professionals and can often recommend salons and hairstylists. These are just a few ideas to help you compile your list.

Once you have four or five candidates, your goal is to visit each salon and to get inside long enough to analyze the surroundings *with your own Close-up Portrait in mind.*

You can tell a great deal about the level of work done at a salon in just one or two minutes, and you should be able to get some feeling for whether your Close-up Portrait stands a chance of getting the right treatment in any particular salon. If the salon looks promising, or if the reception area is totally separate from the working area and you can't tell very much, go ahead and book a manicure in order to further check the place out. Having the manicure in a salon with potential is an inexpensive way to get a good look at the goings-on. Ask the manicurist who is considered the top hairstylist in the establishment, and ask her to point him or her out. Try to get a look at the heads the stylist is working on. A regular manicure (no fancy nail extensions or porcelain nails) runs about six or eight dollars in most salons as of this writing, so you could conceivably execute the manicure gambit in two or three salons without breaking into Junior's college savings account.

While you are comparison shopping, work on your clip file. That cliché "one picture is worth a thousand words" is never truer than when you are conferring with your hairstylist. Develop a collection of photographs to help you communicate your hairstyling needs. As you develop your own gallery of styles, make a note of the ones that you just *hate* as well as those you like. Note pros and cons, find examples if possible, and share these feelings with your hairstylist.

Good clip file sources for:

THE TRULY NATURAL BEAUTY
AND THE CASUAL BEAUTY:
Family Circle
Woman's Day
Good Housekeeping
Self

DESIGNING BEAUTIES:
Vogue
Harper's Bazaar
"W"

ALLURING BEAUTIES:
Cosmopolitan
Glamour

CONTEMPORARY BEAUTIES:
Glamour
Mademoiselle
Working Woman
Self
Harper's Bazaar

AGELESS BEAUTIES:
Vogue
Harper's Bazaar
Glamour ⎫ to keep that
Mademoiselle ⎬ young point
⎭ of view

Day 2—Beauty Essence Workout: Picture Yourself Beautiful

Yesterday you learned to guide your mind toward a successful makeover through the use of positive inner dialogue. Today, I want to explain why pictures are another way to motivate and stimulate the inner beauty essence that will make your outer beauty a reality.

The mind thinks in pictures and will work to make our inner imaginings come true in outer reality. As you build your clip file for your perfect Close-up hairstyle, be on the lookout for photographs of another sort.

See if you can find photographs that embody your beauty essence— evocative perfume ads or editorial photos designed to create a mood are good sources. Also look for photographs of models or celebrities who have some physical similarity to you. Of course, we're simply looking for types here, a message that says "I want to project the visual impact of this picture," whether it be polished and sophisticated, glamorous and alluring, or ageless and elegant. After all, the subconscious mind is suggestible but it's no fool. If you are petite, short and dark, poring over hundreds of pictures of Farrah Fawcett will not turn you into a lanky, angular blonde. *Select photographs that seem to express the best that you want to be.* Once you have started your collection, don't keep it hidden in a folder. Put these photos out where you can see them often, perhaps pasted up around your makeup mirror.

Let these photographs help you practice what Denis Waitley calls "simulation": the neat thing about the brain is that it really is a mimic of what we put into it in advance. Airline pilots have been using simulation for years. So have businesspeople and athletes, who use simulation to experience in their imaginations the games they know they're capable of playing. Actors and actresses call this technique "rehearsal." They create the performance first in their imaginations. So start now to use your photographs to help you experience your beauty essence. This rehearsal will have several positive effects on the success of your makeover.

1. Developing an inner awareness of your beauty goals will reprogram your subconscious, encouraging you to practice and put into effect each step in your Close-up Makeover. Imprinting a specific picture of your beauty ideal on your inner eye *will make your outer beauty a reality.*

2. By picturing yourself beautiful in advance, you will be prepared for it when you achieve it. Waitley explains the importance of rehearsing for success. "We don't spend enough time thinking about how good it is going to feel to be successful. For whatever reason we become successful, we don't completely understand it. And because of this, we don't feel deserving of it. It comes upon us like instant stardom or winning the sweepstakes. Right away our self-talk begins to tear down the success and we get back to where we were before or we go back to being our 'practiced selves.'"

Remember, beauty does start from within. Study your rehearsal pictures daily. Then close your eyes for a second or two and picture yourself as you want to be, as you are going to be, at the successful completion of your Close-up Makeover. Picture yourself beautiful—and you *are!*

Six

DAY THREE

Your Eyebrows

Now you can see why I start makeovers head-first! Your flattering hair color focuses attention on your best features. Your skin tone is noticeably radiant and ready for a new makeup plan, and your eyes especially will take on new drama and color. And interestingly, the frame of beautiful hair focuses attention on your eyebrows, so they are the next important feature that we'll work on.

Why do these two lines play such a major role in your Close-up? They are so important because they can make you look old or young, happy, sad, intelligent or foolish. If you've studied stage makeup, you know how eyebrow placement can totally dominate facial expression. That's why it's essential to have eyebrows that frame your eyes beautifully and express your Close-up Portrait accurately. Objectivision and your Eye-Q Isolation Mask will help you accomplish this.

Analyzing the Role of Brows in Your Close-up

Have you ever taken a small print or photograph and made it appear larger and more important by the frame that you chose? In the same way, eyebrows can enhance, enlarge or correct the shape of the eyes. Since eyebrows and their shape and placement can add nuances of expression to the face, it is very important that the shape itself be a neutral or classic one.

Perhaps women make so many mistakes with their eyebrows because they don't recognize that far from being just two little lines above the eyes, eyebrows consist of three design elements:

- Placement in relation to the eye
- Shape of the brow itself
- Color of the brow

Eyebrows have three design elements:

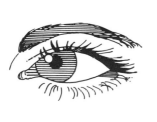 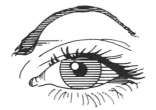 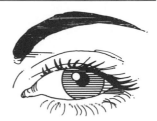

Placement in relation to eye. This brow rides low, crowds the eye.

Shape of the brow itself. Notice how far this "comma" shape is from the ideal gull-wing.

Color. Unless you are a true brunette, too-dark brows can dominate your face, overpower delicate eye color.

While distinctive eyebrows can add impact and pizazz to a face, most women will find that *variations* on the classic brow theme will be most flattering to their expressive eyes.

Before you get busy with tweezers and pencil, decide what you're going to do. Analyze the placement of your brows. Is one brow higher than the other? Objectivision (looking at the reflection of your reflection) should make eyebrow placement very obvious to you. At the same time, decide which of your brows is most attractive in terms of shape and placement, and do all of your shaping and penciling on this one brow.

Next, look directly into the hand mirror and check the placement of your eyebrows in relation to your eyes. They should be at least an eye width (approximately three-quarters to one inch) above your eye. If you've checked your brows and found they are attractively arched above those beautiful orbs of yours, don't be too sure. The majority of women do not see their eyebrows with true Objectivision because, when they look in the mirror to check out their eyebrows or apply makeup, they raise their brows. When they turn away from the mirror, foreheads relaxed, their brows may well slide down to a position unattractively close to the eye.

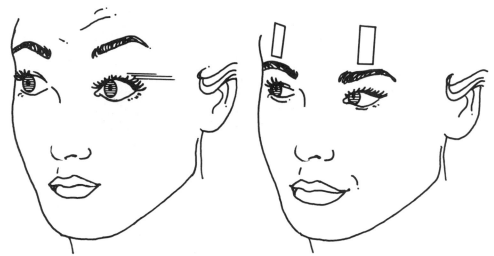

To analyze your eyebrows accurately, correct this hair-raising habit!

To correct this hair-raising habit, apply a strip of Scotch tape vertically from each eyebrow arch up to the hairline. Be sure that your forehead is relaxed when you apply the tape. *Now* look at the true placement of your eyebrows. Perhaps you see that your brows are too close to your eyes, crowding that proportion, making your eyes look smaller than they should.

Next, place your Eye Isolation Mask over your hand mirror. Without your other features to divert your attention, analyze the shape of your

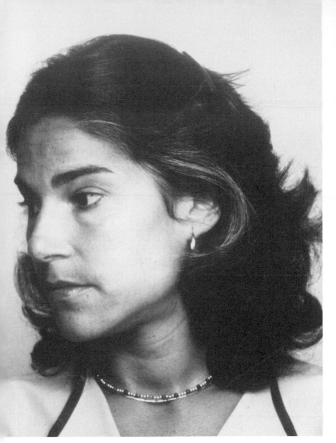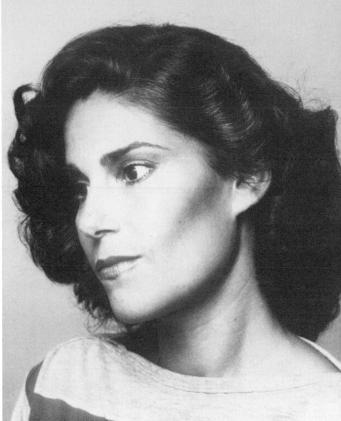

The classic "gull-wing" eyebrow shape is flattering to almost everyone.

eyebrows. Are they too thick? Too thin? Straight and shapeless? If you are using eyebrow pencil, are you aware of a penciled, crayon line? If you can see it, so can other people, and that's not the idea at all.

Look at your brows with sharpened Objectivision and recognize that the delicate eyebrow line is created by individual eyebrow hairs. Can you see the direction the hairs grow? You will repeat this pattern when and if you use eyebrow pencil.

We live in a beauty era when distinctive eyebrows are a definite beauty plus. Still, just as the ideal facial shape is oval, I believe that the classic gull-wing eyebrow shape is the most flattering to the majority of women. As you can see above, this is a brow that is thicker from the inner end to the arch and then tapers out to a thinner line at the outer tip. We use this shape not as an ironclad pattern but rather as a guide to help you create the most flattering brows possible.

Creating Your Ideal Close-up Eyebrows

First, collect the following equipment:
Tweezers
Two eye pencils, one to match eyebrow color, one a few shades
lighter
Translucent powder
Pencil sharpener
Small six-inch ruler
Brow comb and brush
Moustache wax (if brows are luxuriant)
Then follow this procedure to create the perfect brow for your Close-up:

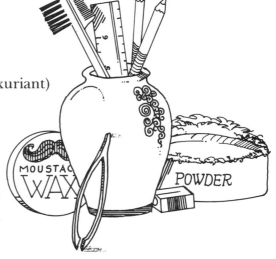

Creating your ideal Close-up brow is easy with the right beauty tools.

1. Remove all traces of eyebrow pencil if you wear it—start with a clean slate.

2. Powder eyebrow area lightly to help you see your brows with Objectivision.

3. Hold the small ruler vertically and line it up with the tear duct. At the spot where the ruler crosses your brow line, make a small dot with the eyebrow pencil (point A).

4. Again, holding the ruler vertically and looking straight ahead, place the ruler at the outer edge of the iris and make a mark where it crosses your eyebrow (point B, the eyebrow arch).

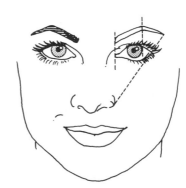

Guide to your Close-up brow line.

SPOT ANNOUNCEMENT

BE SURE THAT YOU USE THE IRIS, THE COLORED PORTION OF
YOUR EYE, INSTEAD OF THE PUPIL, THE BLACK DOT IN THE
CENTER, AS YOUR MEASURING POINT.

5. Place the ruler on a diagonal, lining it up with the nostril and the outer corner of the eye. Your eyebrow should end where the ruler crosses the brow line. Make a dot with the eyebrow pencil (point C). *It is essential that point C should always be higher than point A.* Use the small ruler in a horizontal line between point A and point C to check that your eyebrows do not droop at the end.

6. To ensure that wide-eyed camera-ready look, be sure that your brows are at least an eye width above your eye. Here's how. Hold your ruler vertically and measure the width of your eye from top to bottom at the widest point. Probably an inch wide, more or less. Using this measurement as your guide, mark points A, B and C. Now, connect points A, B and C using the lighter of your two eyebrow pencils. This line

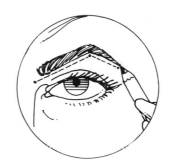

Place guide line at the lower edge of eyebrow.

will be the bottom of the eyebrow shape. To review: point A should start just above the tear duct, a placement that opens your eyes and makes them appear larger; point B, the high point of the eyebrow arch, will give your contours a lift; point C, always higher than point A, also gives the facial contours a lift.

You should have a very clear picture of the ideal and most flattering eyebrow shape for your eyes and how your own eyebrows fit into this pattern. Depending on the thickness of your eyebrow, there will be three ways of creating the most flattering shape.

• If your brows are very thick and heavy, you need a real pruning job. Beauty salons use wax to shape extremely heavy brows, and if you have two fuzzy little caterpillars nestled above your eyes, treat yourself to a waxing. Then faithfully tweeze out the daily crop of eyebrow hairs that will grow back. If you decide to do this job yourself, there are two ways to make it easy. Use a warm wash cloth to soften the skin and make the hair easier to tweeze out (be careful not to smear the eyebrow pattern that you have drawn). Or, if you are very sensitive in the eyebrow area, use an ice cube to slightly numb the skin where you will be tweezing.

● Medium-thick brows should be shaped by tweezing out slipshod offenders, those hairs that detract from the gull-wing eyebrow shape. Also, some delicate penciling may be necessary to augment thin or non-existent hairs. Start first by tweezing hairs that should be removed. Next, alternately using the dark and light eyebrow pencils, fill in the places where your brow doesn't follow our ideal shape using short, hairlike strokes. *Remember that the entire eyebrow contour is created by many, many individual hairs. Any shaping that you do must be created by penciled-in hair lines.*

● The delicate eyebrow. Some women simply have skimpy eyebrows, either from vigorous tweezing or just the natural design of their features. If you have almost no eyebrow hairs, there is a solution. You must become an artist at creating a believable brow through the practiced use of eyebrow pencils. I say *you must* because a nonexistent or too indistinct eyebrow will rob your face of expression and make you look older. The secret of success is, naturally, rehearsal. Practice drawing in a flattering eyebrow arch created by many individual eyebrow hair lines drawn alternately using the two shades of eyebrow pencil. Draw the tiny lines in the direction that your own eyebrow hairs grow.

We've now worked on the placement of your brows and the shape. The next thing to consider is color. This important but often overlooked element in your Close-up will dramatically enhance the beauty of your eyes. We all know that black eyebrow pencil is a no-no. Even if you have very dark brown skin and black hair, do not use black eyebrow pencil. But beyond that injunction, women seem unaware of the many grada-tions of color possible in eyebrow pencils and also in the color of their eyebrows themselves. Shop for pencils that will enhance your personal color scheme. Warm brown, grayed brown, gray, light brown—there are many shades to choose from. You simply have to look.

And while I'm on the subject of eyebrow pencils, remember, less is better. Don't use any at all if you can help it. When in doubt, go toward the lighter shade, as in hair coloring. In fact, even though we are currently in a fashion era where bold brows are "in," it's been my experience that lighter, more delicate brows are flattering to most women, makes one's eyes the focal point of the face, as they should be.

To soften the effect of eyebrow pencil, try this never-fail trick. After you have completed shaping and penciling your brow, powder it. You'll be amazed at how this softens the pencil accents, making them look totally natural, and "sets" the eyebrow line.

If your brows are naturally thick, dark and very emphatic, you can do three things. First, thin out those overpowering brows as the Hollywood pros do by simply tweezing hairs here and there in the body of the brow to soften the impact of its luxuriant growth. Second, you may powder over your brows using a lighter brown shade of powdered eye shadow. This can be a tricky effect in rainstorms so shop until you find an eye shadow that has a very clinging texture. Third, and this is my personal favorite, you can bleach your brows using the mild facial bleach that is available at any drugstore for this purpose. *Do not use hair coloring bleach of any sort to lighten your brows.* The bleach that I've recommended will soften and lighten your brows just a few shades for a very natural believable effect. Or you might consider having your brows bleached at a beauty salon. Again, this can be done for a very nominal fee, and the beauty impact for you is terrific (yes, your eyebrows will grow back in the natural color).

So far, you have been working on the more attractive brow. Once you have perfected it, pencil in the less attractive brow to match. You have now created a flattering basic brow line for yourself. But the goal of your Close-up is to bring out your individual beauty essence, so let's take one final step.

Design Refinements

Again, look at your total face keeping in mind the design themes you have identified through Objectivision. Using your eyebrow pencils to add, or tweezers to subtract, carefully shape eyebrows into a more angular or rounded shape as indicated by the design theme of your face. It creates width in a long narrow face by lengthening the end of your brows a smidge. Instead of placing the peak of your brow (point B) just above the iris, shape the arch a little to the outside of the iris. And note that a low eyebrow arch will also visually widen your facial shape.

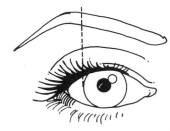

Create the illusion of width in a narrow face by placing peak of brow closer to hairline.

Is your facial theme one of width? Add a lift to your brows at the arch. A high arch will give your face more length.

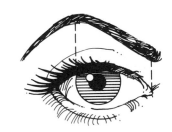

Give your wide face a hint of length by lifting brow arch.

Keep a sense of proportion. Large faces can carry strong, full eyebrow lines. Delicate, fragile faces are overpowered by heavy brows. These variations on a theme must be subtle to be truly effective, but that doesn't mean they are not important. The effectiveness of your Close-up Makeover lies in these kinds of small, easy-to-do details that add up to the total impact. We'll be adding these little design refinements throughout your makeover.

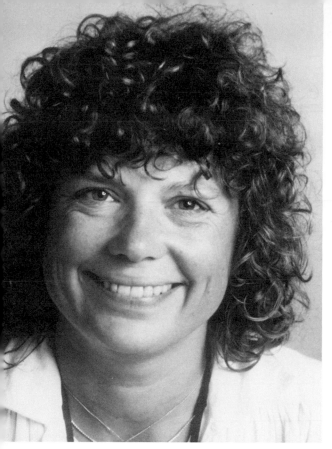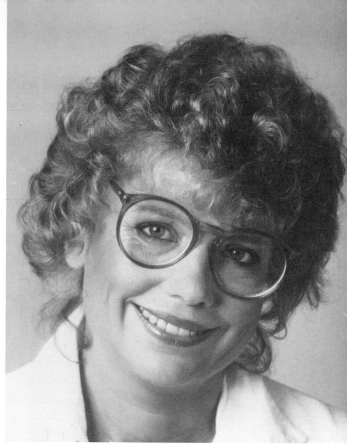

Glasses frames that ride above your brows will give your face a lift.

Eyeglasses

If eyebrows serve to define and accent the beauty of your eyes, eyeglasses create this effect with double impact. Even the most delicate pair will make a bold, strong design statement. They can make your face look wider or longer, your eyes look small or large, and even enhance or detract from the shape of your nose.

Choosing eyeglass frames can be a traumatic experience. Display cases full of those zillions of frames can make it seem impossible to find the one right frame for you. It may help if you realize that you only need one perfect pair to wear all the time. Granted, the fantasy of having a wardrobe of eyeglass frames to suit every mood is an appealing bit of advice from the fashion magazines. But realistically, at today's prices, one perfect pair should be your goal. The following are some shopping tips to help you in your quest.

SHAPE

Let's talk first about glasses in relation to your eyebrows. A standard bit of advice is, "One set of eyebrows is all you need, so be sure that the eyeglass frames cover your eyebrows." That *sounds* reasonable, but in actual practice when women wear eyeglasses that are on a line with their natural brow, the effect of the eyeglasses is to drag down all of the facial contours. If you wear glasses, try this and see for yourself. Lift your frames up just a tad, so that they are just above your natural brow line. Can you see how that miraculously gives your entire face a lift? True, if you have heavy dark brows and heavy dark eyeglass frames, you will create the impression of double trouble in the eyebrow department. But choosing frames that cover your dark brows and thereby lower all of your facial contours is not the solution. Rather, if you have heavy brows, choose a rimless, light eyeglass frame that rides above your brows and gives your face that magical lift.

Another design blooper is that eyeglasses very often ride too low on the cheek contour and repeat the shape or color of under-eye circles or bags. Bad news. If your frames break either of these design rules, seriously consider replacing them with one that will be as wildly flattering as your first great love.

● Oval faces can get away with just about any shape or any size of glasses.

● If your face is round, choose frames that are narrow vertically but wide horizontally—for example, an oval shape. Incidentally, short pudgy noses look better in frames without nose pads which tend to visually "fatten" the bridge of the nose.

● Short square faces look best in enormous round eyeglass frames or rectangular shapes in which the lower outside corners extend out over the cheekbone, thus cutting the width of the jawline and making the face appear more oval. Frames that sit up on the nose, not on the cheek bone, will elongate the look of the face.

● Long faces need deep wide frames that cover a good portion of the face and thus shorten it. Enormous round glasses are also good for this

Eyeglass frames to flatter: _____

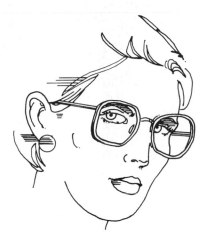

Oval faces _____

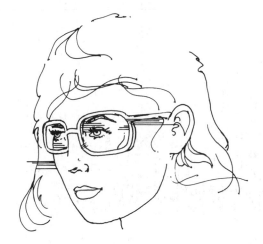

Round faces _____

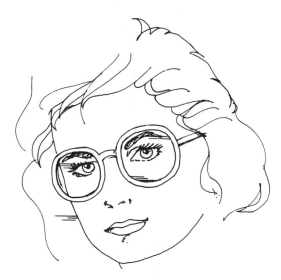

Square faces _____

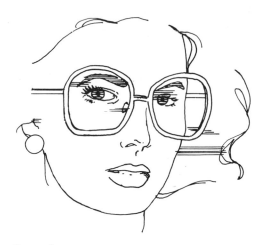

Long faces _____

design theme. Long noses look shorter if the bridge of the frame sits partially down on the nose.

COLOR

Hair color and eye color are two considerations in choosing the frame color that will be most flattering to you. If you want to accent your eye color, this is a cardinal rule: choose eyeglass frames in a soft muted shade similar to your eye color, but not matching it. Remember, the natural tones throughout the face are delicate and easily overpowered by man-made color schemes. In other words, if you have blue eyes, do not choose bright blue frames—select softly muted smoky blue glasses. By contrast your eyes will appear very blue.

If you choose frames to blend with your hair color, your choices again are rather obvious.

- Blonde hair: sable, light shell, even metallic gold frames
- Brunette: medium to dark tortoise shell, faux bamboo wooden frames
- Redheads: all the tawny shades from champagne to sherry
- Silver hair: platinum, silver, gray, metallic

GLASSES AND YOUR CLOSE-UP PORTRAIT

Truly Natural Beauties: Benjamin Franklin steel frames, "Aunt Polly" nose-perchers.

Casual Beauties: Sporty, racy shapes, i.e., pilot's glasses. Also brightly colored plastic frames: bright red or bright blue, for example.

Contemporary Beauties: Weighty, powerful frames in medium to dark colors. Careful here. Studious, bookkeeper frames are not the image you want at all. Some younger Contemporary Beauties or those with very fragile delicate features may choose nonprescription eyeglasses simply for the power impact of a strong, heavy frame.

Designing Beauties: Because glasses can make such a fashion statement, you may invest in a wardrobe of designer glasses, matching color and texture with your various outfits. Note: extreme designs in eyeglass frames go out of fashion as rapidly as extreme designs in clothing items. Can your budget take it?

Alluring Beauties: Delicate, rimless eyeglass frames enhance your feminine image. Pearl blue or lilac-tinted lenses will give your eyes a melting appeal.

Ageless Beauties: Bold, fashionable, dramatic glasses that make a design statement will give the mature woman an ageless image. Conservative, ladylike glasses designed to blend into the background and pretend they are not glasses are just plain matronly.

Beautiful eyebrows and flattering glasses will frame your eyes in a look you will love. And this is just the beginning. As you work through your makeover, daily adding those enhancing details that comprise your new image, you will have to deal, increasingly, with another aspect of beauty.

Day 3 — Beauty Essence Workout: Learn to Love Being Looked At!

One of the payoffs of your Close-up Makeover will be this: you're going to get more attention. The thought, time and effort that you put into your Close-up marks you as a Special Woman—and it *shows*. Increasingly, you'll be the object of admiring glances—and quite likely you'll overhear flattering comments ranging from, "Who is that fascinating woman?" to "Wow!" You're looking just fabulous, and people will notice!

Does this news make you feel terrific? Maybe, and maybe not. Many women are unprepared to accept the admiration that is a natural by-product of the Close-up Makeover. If you are not prepared for the positive attention, if you fear it, you may *subconsciously* sabotage your efforts to complete a successful makeover. So it's important to recognize that on some level you may feel discomfort with admiration, and deal with it right now.

Actually, this discomfort is easy to understand. We all carry around a collection of old tapes imprinted by foolish or thoughtless people in our childhood. "Pretty is as pretty does," "Don't try to be something that you're not," "I'm glad to see that you're sensible, not flighty and irresponsible like that beautiful sister of yours." It's important to be aware of these messages and to recognize how inappropriate they are for the confident, beautiful woman you are becoming.

Another cause for discomfort with admiration is that in the process of your Close-up Makeover you are developing new ways of *feeling* about yourself. And anytime we are involved in change, we tend to feel uncertain and vulnerable.

The world of the theater gives us many techniques for dealing with self-consciousness. After all, being an actress means being looked at. But you don't have to be on the stage to benefit from the technique of developing Presence—one that helps you create the self-possessed aura that is the basis of self-confidence.

Self-possessed—what an interesting and accurate term. Self-consciousness literally scatters our energy—our personality essence, if you will. When we are the uneasy object of other people's attention and thus become self-conscious, we usually become conscious of ourselves in a *negative* way. We scatter our attention to multitudes of imagined deficiencies in our bodies, slumping to hide a too-full bust, dipping our heads to negate a too-tall figure, and fumbling with our hands. Also, self-consciousness automatically creates overactive, anxious facial expressions. With our attention thus scattered hither and yon, no wonder we feel uncomfortable. (We don't look so good, either!) But we can recapture a feeling of ease by "collecting ourselves," literally drawing our energy, our sense of self, back to our very center. Here's how.

Close your eyes and place your hand on your solar plexus (that soft muscle area just below your rib cage). Think of this area of your body as a magnet and imagine that you are attracting all of your scattered energy to this center. Why the solar plexus? For some reason this area becomes the focal point of stage fright and self-consciousness. If you've ever had butterflies in your stomach, then you know how true this is. To magically release this feeling of tension, of stage fright or self-consciousness, *slowly* inhale and exhale. Calm and quiet your breathing. Think of pulling that scattered energy into your solar plexus as you inhale.

Of course you will practice this technique until it becomes easy, natural, and unobtrusive. After all, you don't see Raquel Welch or Twiggy standing in the center of a Broadway stage clutching her midsection, closing her eyes, and breathing heavily. Actresses have practiced so that this centering ability is second nature. Well, you must practice too, and make this process of focusing an easy, effortless skill. Believe me, the payoffs are impressive. You will automatically possess *Presence,* that aura of personal power that is the direct result of centering, not scattering, your self-awareness. And, from this calm center, from this assured vantage point, I promise you, you'll *love* being looked at.

Seven

DAY FOUR

Makeup: The Foundation of Your Close-up Portrait

An important part of every scene on TV is the stage set, a carefully calculated and subtly lighted background, designed to create the perfect foundation for star performers. In the same way, your makeup sets the stage for your leading performers, your eyes and lips. Today you will learn how to create this foundation for your Close-up, calling on an ensemble of talented performers to back you up. These performers are (in order of appearance):

1. Moisturizer
2. Makeup base
3. Blusher
4. Sculpturing products (special cameo appearances): highlight and shadow creams, highlight and shadow powders, matte and luster products
5. Powder

Moisturizer — the Understudy

The first thing to know is that your makeup base is always preceded by a moisturizer. One of the triumphs of modern cosmetic laboratories is the infinite variety of truly effective moisturizing products designed to correct and combat almost every skin problem.

There is a menu to suit every skin's appetite and knowledgeable skin technicians at cosmetic counters can direct you to the right product for your complexion. Moisturizers play a specific role in your Close-up Portrait and suggestions for your own best type are outlined in the Close-up Portrait section.

While moisturizers do an infinity of beneficial things to the quality of your skin, let's examine what they do visually, in terms of setting the stage for your eyes and lips. Since the moisturizing lotion smoothes and "plumps" the skin's surface by holding moisture there, this fine lotion film tends to obscure minute structural flaws, fill in the gaps, and stop the scattering of light.

A key point here: whatever moisturizing lotion you choose, be sure to apply it to the *entire* face and neck area, paying special attention to eyelids and to the under-eye area. The lotion fills in and minimizes those tiny expression lines. You can prove it to yourself how very important moisturizers are, visually, by trying this little test. Apply a moisturizer liberally to the back of your right hand, leaving the other in its normal, probably dry, state. Now, fill a puff with translucent powder and pat the back of both hands. Brush excess powder off, and look at both hands.

Wow! Immediately you will see that the left hand, powdered without benefit of moisturizing lotion, looks depressingly like the entire Colorado River Basin in the middle of July—cracks, furrows, crevices and grooves will leap out in appalling detail. Ah, but the skin of the right hand looks just the way skin ought to look: moist, plumped up, smooth and with a natural luster. *That's* why you should always use a moisturizing lotion.

Foundation Plays the Lead in Your Beautiful Close-up

Your makeup base is "as close to carrying a spare skin as a woman will ever get." That's how Marv Westmore describes foundation, this most talented of all cosmetic products. Yet so many women tell me, often with a touch of pride, "Oh, I never wear any makeup at all." I know, I know. It's very obvious that you're not wearing makeup base because it's a one-in-a-million complexion that looks truly beautiful without the aid of this miraculous, and *beneficial,* cosmetic product. So why fight it?

Look at what the right makeup base can do for you:

1. *Protection.* Contemporary makeups are designed to protect the skin from pollution and the drying effects of weather and environment; to lubricate and moisturize the skin; and in some cases to protect it from the ravaging effects of the sun. In other words, today's makeup bases are *good* for your skin.

2. *Color.* Tinted makeup base is the background for your Close-up Portrait and is designed to create a smooth, one-color basis for the rest of your cosmetic ensemble. We are not always conscious of the uneven color quality of our skin, but an application of makeup base immediately shows how attractive a perfect complexion color can be.

3. *Perfect Texture.* Makeup base gives the complexion a fine-textured, poreless look that is the ideal quality of a flawless complexion. This perfect texture also serves as a "prime coat" for all of the other cosmetic items you will be using.

That's what's good about makeup base. What's bad is that incorrectly used it can make a woman look painted, artificial, old, cheap—you name it.

WHAT'S THE PROBLEM? COLOR

Color is the secret of a natural look. Too many women try to add color and vitality to their complexion by choosing a makeup base two or three shades deeper than their own coloring. Almost everything that you don't

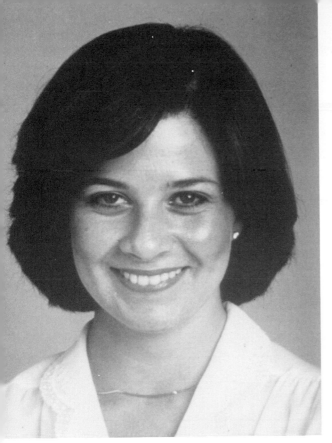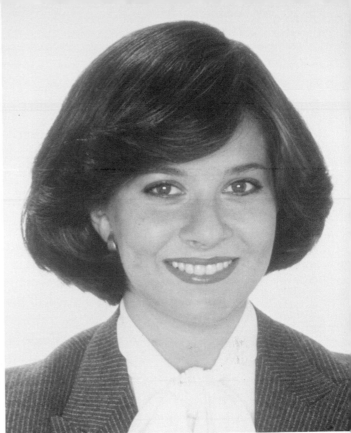

Makeup base creates the perfect foundation for all other cosmetics.

like about makeup can be corrected by choosing a foundation that matches your skin tone *exactly,* or is one shade lighter. Makeup base is the one character in your Close-up cast that must appear to be totally natural. Lipstick and eye makeup can look dramatic or slightly artificial; even blushers can look a bit like makeup or a bit supernatural and still be attractive. But when it comes to makeup base, we can't forgive even a hint of artificiality. Can you see why color is the most important element in your choice of makeup base?

You must have your wits about you when you go to the cosmetic counter to choose your foundation color. This is really one of the most difficult challenges you will face in creating your entire Close-up Portrait. The many color choices in foundation can be confusing. After all, white skin is divided into twelve basic color shades with an infinite variety of gradations in each of the twelve categories. Black skin becomes even more of a challenge; there can be thirty-five basic shadings for black skin with all of the gradations of color for each of the thirty-five. The most common mistake is to try to add color and vitality to your complexion by selecting a shade two or three shades deeper than your own coloring (or, in the case of black women, makeup that is too light). If you choose foundation that matches your skin tone *exactly,* you can't go wrong.

In spite of the infinite number of cosmetic shades available, you may find it difficult to match your skin exactly. Mixing is the solution to this color problem. Choose the two shades that are closest to your own skin tone and mix them. It's also a good idea to have two shades that represent your winter and summer face coloring. The lightest shade, perhaps with some mixing on your part, will be worn in the winter. But as your skin becomes slightly tanned or colored by the spring and summer sun, you can segue into the darker shade by mixing.

Another quality that is essential to a natural look is texture—that luminous, fine-pored, perfect complexion can only be achieved with a makeup base that is right for your skin type. Technically, makeup base comes in several forms: liquid makeup, cream base (a paste or solid tinted foundation sold in jars, compact cakes, or stick form), powder combined with base (a tinted cake of solid face powder). The liquid form is by far the best choice for your overall makeup base. There is a liquid makeup that will be right for your skin type, and it gives the best, most natural-looking coverage with the sheerest texture. You will just have to experiment a bit to find the one that is most flattering to your individual complexion.

HOW TO FIND THE RIGHT MAKEUP BASE FOR YOU

Here is how to shop for your own perfect makeup base. Insist on a "try-on" of every product you are seriously considering. After all, at today's prices your purchase of even a single bottle of makeup base can involve a sizeable amount of money. So sample, and don't be afraid to ask. The first step in your try-on is to apply the makeup base to the back of either hand. You're looking now for texture and coverage. Does the product seem too thick, does it slide away into nothing, do you like the luminous quality? Do you like the way it feels, is it too sticky, too heavy? Once you have narrowed your product choices down to two or three, you're ready to start the serious business of color selection. Apply a dab of each color you are considering onto your jaw line and compare. Seeing them side by side makes color choice easier. You should also scrutinize these shades in several kinds of light because colors will vary.

APPLICATION

This must be an absolutely flawless performance—no streaks, no obvious lines of demarcation, no gaps in the film of foundation covering your face and neck. This demand for perfection may seem difficult and uncompromising but is really very easy to attain. Simply use the one indispensable tool of all professional makeup artists—the makeup sponge.

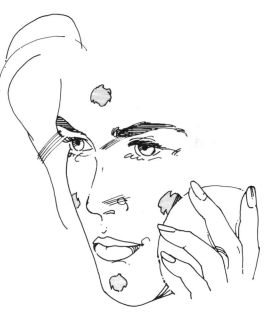

When you apply your foundation makeup, dot it liberally over the face, being sure to put a dot on each eyelid, and then smooth it over your entire face with a makeup sponge, paying special attention to the eye area and the nostrils. Cover the lips thoroughly, patting and smoothing. (Remember, you are not trying to rub the makeup *into* your skin, but rather to smooth and flow it over the surface of your skin.)

Another secret for a flawless performance is to apply makeup base to your earlobes. Smooth the foundation under your jawline so that it blends into the natural shadow formed by your jawbone. By meticulously applying makeup in these areas, you will forever banish

Apply makeup base with a sponge for a flawless finish.

the unattractive and artificial Kabuki mask effect that is so often seen.

Color Up with Blusher

Blusher is *the* indispensable beauty maker. Like the "on" switch of your TV set, it switches on the glow, the vitality, the beauty life in your face. If you were to wear no other makeup, blush would still give your looks a lift.

Lift! That's the secret bonus of blush, the true double-feature cosmetic. In addition to color and glow, the knowledgeable application of blushers can lift and contour your face in an effective and unmistakable way. But perhaps this double bonus is the very reason that so many women use blush incorrectly.

BLUSHING BLOOPERS

Women get confused about the purpose of blush. Is it for color? Is it for contour? The answer is: blush does both. This confusion is reflected in the many mistakes in blusher application that I see. For example:

1. Dark-hued powdered blush, ideal for sculpturing cheekbones, is often used on the high points of cheeks to add color. This either creates a heavy painted look, a flat slab-like cheek contour or, worst of all, an impression of tired sunken cheeks.

2. Either light or dark blush applied too close to the nose makes noses appear larger (horrors!); applied too close to the eyes, it creates a painted, fevered look.

3. In an attempt to create dramatic cheekbones, dark-hued blush is applied in the cheekbone hollow and down onto the lower part of the cheek, creating a gaunt, wasted look.

These visual disasters are caused by putting the wrong colors in the wrong place and are the result of a limited vision of your facial structure. Again, Objectivision comes to the rescue. Once you *see* and understand what you are trying to do, it is very easy to use blushers—or any cosmetic, for that matter—in a super-flattering way.

HOW TO APPLY YOUR BLUSHER

Look into your mirror. Smile, and really study the contours of those soon-to-be rosy cheeks. Your cheek contour is composed of two geometric shapes—the rounded "apples" of your cheeks (directly under your eyes) and a "wedge" of bone that angles up and out toward the top of your ear. Yes, that's the infamous cheekbone upon which so many Hollywood careers have been built. This apple-wedge contour is what you will be coloring and contouring with blushers.

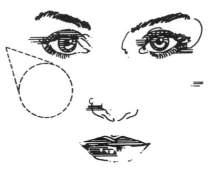

Relax your face and, still looking into the mirror, suck in your cheeks so that the cheekbone hollows are accented. Place your fingers in each cheek hollow. You will be able to feel your teeth through the cheek tissue. Be totally aware of this hollow area because *you will not apply any blusher into this hollow area.* Yes, I know. Fashion models and movie stars seem to, without exception, have a glamorous dark shadow in the lower cheek. You would too if you had a lighting director following you around to be sure that all light sources hit your cheekbones with just the right dramatic effect! But we're talking about real life, and real women have rosy cheeks, not sunken dark hollow ones.

Color and contour the "apple-wedge" area for beautiful cheekbones.

More placement tips:
- Never apply blusher closer to the nose than the center of the eye.
- Never apply blusher up into the eye circle.
- Always apply color *above* the cheekbone hollow.

Of course the edges of the colored blushing area may softly blend out into these spots above and below your apple-wedge contour. But the highest intensity of color will remain in the apple-wedge.

Now let's talk about color. The color intensity of your blusher should be applied in three levels:
- *First level:* the deepest, most intense blush color is applied just above the cheekbone hollow;

Here is your guide to contouring your face with blusher.

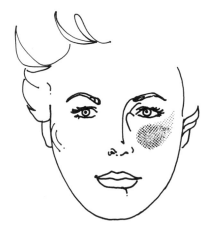

OVAL FACE: *greatest color intensity on "apple" of cheek. Blend color up and out onto wedge.*

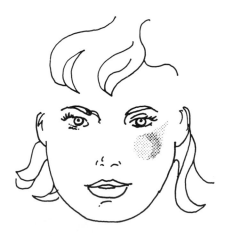

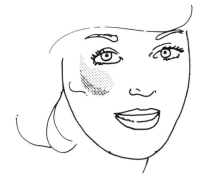

ROUND OR TRIANGULAR FACE: *apply greatest color intensity on outer half of "apple," then blend color up, lifting "wedge," and down over large jaw line.*

OBLONG FACE: *keep intensity of color on lower part of apple-wedge, and accent horizontal placement of color.*

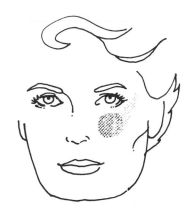

SQUARE, WIDE FACE: blusher angles up to create length. Do not extend color out to hairline. Highest intensity of color is on "apple" of cheeks.

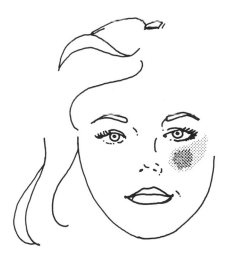

INVERTED TRIANGLE: keep color intensity in middle of apple-wedge contour to deemphasize cheekbone width.

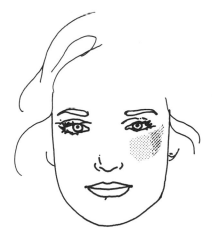

Keep blusher's color intensity away from a "generous" nose.

- *Second level:* the brightest blushing color is applied on the "apple" of the cheek;
- *Third level:* the lightest color just highlights the top of the apple-wedge contour.

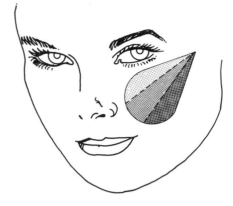

You'll use this three-color approach to shape and contour your face. But first, choose your weapons!

Depending on the product used, blush delivers its color impact in several ways.

- *Matte finish*—powdered blush
- *Moist dewy finish*—creams, gels
- *Polished finish*—liquid blush (sometimes called color wash, usually has pearlescent quality)

Each form of blush has a different effect and different purpose, as I'll be explaining in the Close-up Portrait Gallery.

Sculpturing Your Best Camera Angles

To get an even clearer picture of how sculpturing works, read this next section. Remember, even if you never intend to do the more involved techniques, the *theory* is essential because every time you apply blush to your face, you are visually altering its contours. Incidentally, the theory behind sculpturing is not that difficult. I have the word of my friend Academy-Award-winner William Tuttle, head of makeup at MGM for twenty years. He told me, "Any woman can learn to do a complete sculpturing job and she can do it in about ten minutes." In a lengthy interview, Bill and I discussed basic contouring theory and our approaches to sculpturing techniques. Now I want to share these points with you.

- *Light colors:* accentuate, highlight or enlarge an area
- *Dark colors:* minimize or reduce an area

Through the use of light enlargers and dark reducers, the face as a whole and individual features can be brought into better and more harmonious proportion. The light and dark cosmetic products used can be broken down further as to their visual effects: lustrous products will reflect light and accent an area; matte finishes, because they do not reflect light, de-emphasize an area; warm tones (in blushers) will accent an area and make it look larger; cool tones (blue-based reds) will reduce an area and make it look smaller.

Sculpturing products come in a variety of forms:

- Cover sticks in light or dark shades
- Translucent creams or liquids in light shades
- Foundation: two shades lighter or two shades darker than your overall face makeup
- Powder: pearlescent highlight powder or shadowing powder, two shades darker than your overall foundation

Opaque products are applied *under* your overall foundation. Translucent products are patted *over* your foundation color. Light and dark powders are dusted on after all makeup elements are completed.

- Products for sculpturing large areas (forehead, cheeks, jaw, chin):
    Light foundation
    Dark foundation
    Light powder
    Dark powder
    Blushers
- Products for sculpturing small areas (the eye area, nose, upper lip, small hollows and lines):
    Light/dark opaque cover sticks
    Light/dark translucent creams
    Liquid pearlescent highlighters

The drawing on the next page will give you an idea of where to use these light and dark products.

Now let's relate this to your face. Using Objectivision technique #1,

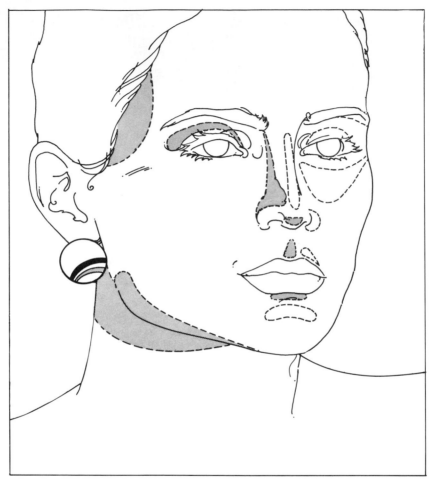

Sculpture beautiful contours through the magic of light and shadow.

SPOT ANNOUNCEMENT

WOMEN WITH DARK SKINS WILL FIND THAT ALL KINDS OF LIGHT SCULPTURING PRODUCTS WILL HELP THEM ACCENT BONE STRUCTURE, CALLING ATTENTION TO BEST FEATURES. DARK CONTOURING IS USUALLY LESS SUCCESSFUL ON DARK SKIN. BUT REMEMBER, BLUSHERS WILL GIVE EVERY WOMAN A FAST AND EASY WAY TO SCULPTURE BEAUTIFUL CAMERA-READY PROPORTIONS.

draw the outline of your face on your makeup mirror. Then mark on the mirror the planes of your face that you wish to lift or enlarge, and those areas you wish to reduce. (Remember, *keep one eye closed* as you draw.) Use light and dark cover sticks or two shades of lipstick. Sharpen your Objectivision awareness by being specific in these markings. You know your facial shape and the themes of your face by now, so don't just look. See! Should your cheekbone highlight angle *up*, to create length on your wide face? Or should the highlight (and yes, blusher) go directly to the *side*, creating horizontal impact in your long facial proportions?

When you complete your sculpturing analysis, take a clean piece of typing paper, press it against the mirror to transfer your unique sculpture pattern onto the paper. Using this Objectivision pattern to help you, complete your sculpturing analysis.

CAMOUFLAGING UNDER-EYES

Now, I want to give you some detailed pointers on camouflaging eyebags and circles because almost every woman has to deal with one of these problems. Eyebags can be a special trial. I see so many women misuse cover sticks, actually accenting eyebags, and turning them into attention-getters!

Dark circles under the eyes can be covered with your light sculpture products. There are several ways to do this as outlined in the various Close-up Portraits. But bags under the eyes present more of a challenge.

The sculpturing principle here is to highlight the sunken circle and shadow the prominent bag right above it thereby giving the illusion of a smooth, lifted contour to the entire eye area. Apply highlighting foundation or cover stick over the hollow or darkened circle under the eye. Pat gently

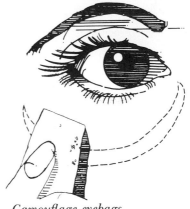

Camouflage eyebags with this highlight and shadowing technique.

and thoroughly. Next, apply dark foundation over the puffy area which rises directly above the sunken eye circle. The principle here is to highlight the sunken circle and shadow the prominent fullness right above it. It is essential to blend thoroughly—using your indispensable makeup sponge—so there is no line of demarcation where these two colors come together.

Sculpturing your face to create the most beautiful proportions possible is a basic element in all makeup plans. But how much sculpturing you do and with what products will be dictated by your Close-up Portrait. Look now at your Close-up Portrait for the step-by-step plan to help you create the foundation for your right face.

Makeup for Your Close-up Portrait

TRULY NATURAL BEAUTIES

You never wear foundation, seldom blusher ("I just pinch my cheeks a couple of times—it gives such a natural look") and even go without moisturizer. The message is "What you see is what you get." But listen, TNBs, so many of you aren't really seeing yourselves in relation to the world that you live in. Running wild and free along the sands of Big Sur may indeed add vitality and color to your complexion, but the truth is that many, many TNBs work in urban settings with twentieth-century machines rather than in bucolic settings at a hand loom or potter's wheel. So I urge you to use some type of moisturizer as protection.

A trip to your favorite health food store will reveal many truly natural products that not only look natural but contribute to the health of your complexion as well. Moisturizers containing aloe vera are especially beneficial. And if you spend a great deal of time outdoors, look for products that contain the B-vitamin PABA, which is a natural sunscreen. Incidentally, if you hate to put anything on your face, it may be because you have an allergy to one of the most common ingredients used in all makeups—glycerin. When I work with women and hear comments like: "I hate makeup—it feels as if my skin can't breathe," or "The moment I put makeup on, I know it's there and I can't forget it," I feel sure that these women have a makeup allergy. Moisturizers and makeup without glycerin are not easy to find, so read labels carefully. One glycerin-free moisturizer that I can recommend is available from Reviva Labs (705 Hopkins Road, Haddonfield, NJ 08033).

What about sculpturing your face to enhance your best features and minimize those that are less perfect? I have no directions for you in this category because the very idea of camouflage seems dishonest to your idealistic concept of beauty. Of course, when you want to express the more worldly side of your nature, you can refer to other more sophisticated portraits—the Designing Beauty or the Alluring Beauty.

Now, about those rosy cheeks. The biggest beauty problem for TNBs is a lack of color. It's a sad contradiction of the beauty ideal of glowing health, but the unadorned face almost always looks pale, wan, and under par in contemporary lighting. A little face color does wonders to create that look of carefree, gimmick-free honesty that you admire. A perfect product for this purpose is called "Indian Earth," a naturally occurring "mixture of minerals existing in oxide silicate and carbonate forms as they occur in nature." How natural can you get? You'll love this earth-tone powder in its little hand-made pot. It can be dusted across the cheeks, used to add a natural color to your lips, and even dabbed on the eyelids for a natural eyeshadow. Create a healthy apple-cheeked look by smiling at yourself in the mirror and lightly brushing this powder onto the high points of your cheeks and across the bridge of your nose. You can also give your face the look of a bronzed sun goddess: mix a touch of the magic bronze powder with your moisturizer, blend in the palm of your hand, and smooth this liquid sunshine onto your forehead just below the hairline, on the tip of your chin, and on your earlobes.

THE CASUAL BEAUTY

Your breezy, on-the-go image will get some needed polish with makeup and blushers, but time is of the essence in your life, so here are some speedy plans that work perfectly for your lifestyle.

1 *Moisturizers/foundation.* Many cosmetic lines have a tinted moisturizer. These products combine moisturizer and sheer foundation in one easily applied step. In addition, these products may also have a sunscreen, an essential ingredient for you active Casual Beauties.

2 *Sculpturing.* "Are you kidding? Who has time?" You're absolutely right. But remember, the moment you put blusher on your cheeks you are creating sculpturing effects. So reread the section on blushers as sculpturing elements, and don't waste time by just slapping that color on your face. Do it right and make every beauty gesture count.

If you have under-eye circles, you may be tempted to use a concealer, but any opaque product will be too obvious in the intense, outdoor light. First of all, be aware that your dark circles will be less noticeable in sunlight because of the play of light and shadows on your face. However, if you still feel that you have a real problem, simply use a light shade of foundation, close to your skin tone. Apply in the circle area after you have applied your tinted moisturizer. Pat, pat, pat to blend.

3 *Blusher.* Give your cheeks a natural glow with a gel stick, a sheer gel blusher that looks like a fat-and-sassy lipstick tube. Not only can you stroke on color in a jiffy, but the giant gel tube is easy to carry and slips conveniently into the bottom of a jogging or tennis bag. Since sunshine intensifies all colors, choose your gel blush in a light red or pink shade, colors that look perfectly natural in the bright sun and tend to mimic your own sun-kissed flush of color.

4 *Powder.* Whether in the form of blush or face powder, this is definitely a no-no when you're spending time outdoors. It will look chalky and artificial, and if your complexion has a healthy gleam, that's just the image for you outdoor Casual Beauties. But if your super-oily complexion is more grease than gleam, keep a supply of those little blotters called "Face Savers" (available at any drugstore) to soak up excess oils.

CONTEMPORARY BEAUTIES

It's essential that your complexion project an image of dynamic energy. But those villainous fluorescent lights ever-present in the workplace can give the healthiest skin a cold, harsh appearance. A few take-charge makeup tricks will solve this problem.

1 *Moisturizer.* Unless your skin is very oily, consider a super-lubricating moisturizer to counteract dry office air.

2 *Sculpturing.* Fluorescent lighting intensifies under-eye shadows, so most working women will need a good opaque shadow cover for the under-eye area. Since fluorescent lighting has bluish-green overtones, look for a shadow cover in a pink or peachy shade rather than clear white. Use this opaque shadow cover to accent or create a good, strong, determined jawline. Or use two shades of foundation makeup to sculpture your face, diminishing soft contours, accenting strong determined ones.

3 *Foundation.* Choose a makeup base with a matte finish rather than a light-reflective one—much more flattering under those dreadful lights. And choose a base with a peachy rather than pink tone.

4 *Blusher.* To maintain that look of healthy vitality all day long, your blushing plan comes in two parts. Start with a liquid gel that comes in a tube. Apply with a makeup sponge, pat and blend. You'll find that these gel blushers last and last. But you can rev up the color throughout the day with a powdered blush in a related color that will continue the matte-finish theme. Now, about colors for your blusher. Those quirky fluorescent lights cause havoc with all red tones, so avoid them. The most effective way of counteracting the debilitating visual effects of fluorescent lighting is to use a tone-on-tone color scheme. Choose a warm golden, apricot or coral shade for your gel blush. For smooth coverage, apply with a makeup sponge while your foundation is still slightly damp. Then, intensify cheek color during the day with a powdered blush that has a touch of pink in it. This tone-on-tone effect gives a dot of rosy color that can stand up to those ghastly fluorescent lights.

5 *Powder.* For touch-ups during the day and to keep the velvety matte finish that is so flattering for Contemporary Beauties, use pressed powder (so easy to slide a little compact into a desk drawer). The trick is to apply it with a Big Daddy brush. This effect lasts and lasts and it's fast too. Incidentally, black beauties should choose powder in a shade darker than their skin tone since powder products tend to turn ashen on dark skin.

DESIGNING BEAUTIES

You were the first to know that makeup not only makes you look good but can also be good for you. You have followed with fascination as the cosmetic industry developed treatment products, moving from vitamins to collagen/elastin moisturizers and finally to the latest development— the cell-renewal systems that are part of every leading cosmetic company's line. Casual Beauties may scoff and say "it all comes out of one barrel," but you've done your homework and know that a moisturizer can work all day like a friendly genie to create skin-renewing miracles underneath your makeup.

1 *Moisturizer.* You'll be wearing the latest beauty breakthrough.

2 *Sculpturing.* Designing Beauties are devoted to the art of makeup and use a palette of highlight and shadow products to design their most flattering face. Here is one plan that I would call "the works." You will need the following products:

- Opaque cover stick highlight
- Translucent peachy cream highlight
- 20-30-40 cream shadow (available through William Tuttle Custom Color Cosmetics, Frenchy Beauty Supply Company, 5202 Laurel Canyon Blvd., North Hollywood, CA 91607) for modeling small areas—forehead, under the chin, the delicate planes of the nose
- Foundation two shades darker than your makeup base

A. Use opaque shadow cover stick to really lift up small indented areas (eye circles, laugh lines, etc.). This product can also be used to give emphasis to delicate bone structure in this way: apply a wedge of opaque cover-up at the high point of your cheekbone near the temple; or if cheeks are flat, start the opaque wedge directly under the iris and blend out and up toward the temple. Instant cheekbones! And flattering to any facial shape.

B. Apply foundation makeup, blending with a makeup sponge. Be sure to smooth the makeup base over any opaque cover-up areas. Do not try to rub the foundation into your skin, thus spoiling your sculpturing. Rather, think of layering the foundation makeup easily over opaque cover-up.

C. Working quickly while your makeup base is still damp, blend the darker foundation shade over large areas that you wish to diminish, for example, a too-wide jawline, double chin, or protruding forehead. Remember, blend your two shades of base as thin and smooth as silk. This darker foundation technique is also great for diminishing the sides of a too-broad nose or the tip of a nose that's a bit too long. Blended properly, this shadow sculpturing defies detection.

D. Now, use the 20-30-40 cream (or any dark cream) to reduce and indent small contours, to narrow the bridge of the nose near the eye, to model generous nostrils, to create a shadow under the lower lip, to eliminate that stubborn little pad of fat directly under the chin.

E. Translucent peachy cream is used to further lift and accent the high points of the face.

3 *Blusher.* A trio of blushers will create—or enhance—high-fashion cheekbones.

A. Apply translucent apricot or pink liquid blush in a soft wash of color on the "apple" of cheeks, blending with your sponge out to hairline and up toward the temples.

B. Sweep powder blush in a plum or bronze shade *just above* the cheekbone hollow. You Designing Beauties know that this placement lifts contours, at the same time creating the illusion of prominent cheekbones.

C. Finally, powdered blush in a light, luminous shade of apricot or pink is applied just above the dark blush—and blended so that no line of demarcation is visible.

4 *Powder.* While others use powder simply to "set" makeup and create a matte finish, you continue your creative contouring magic by using light, luminous powder to further emphasize cheek bones and jaw line, or to straighten the bridge of your nose. A darker shade (carefully chosen so that it contains *no* red tones) is brushed just under your jaw line and may shadow the tip of a too-long nose.

THE ALLURING BEAUTY

The face of the Alluring Beauty is luminous and softly rosy. Since you are so often viewed across a cozy table for two lit with warm glowing candles, or in a quiet room aglow with subdued incandescent lighting, you are an expert at creating a makeup that looks glamorous yet natural in these romantic settings. For daytime makeup, take your color cues from other Close-up Portraits.

1 *Moisturizer.* You love the "dewy" look and give your face a spritz of Evyan water before applying a rich moisturizer.

2 *Contouring.* You will create softly rounded cheeks and chin with opaque light cover sticks. Two highlight dots on the upper lip directly above the cupid's bow will make your mouth more shapely and accent that appealing dimple in your upper lip. A touch of dark contour cream just under your lower lip will create a provocative pout!

3 *Foundation.* Choose a softly pearlized, light-reflecting foundation that will give your face a luminous moon goddess look in dim light.

4 *Blusher.* Romantic lighting has golden overtones, so coral, peach, bronze and other warm-toned blushers will be especially flattering. Use powdered luminous blush in three tones, for example, amber just above the cheekbone hollow, peach on the fullest part of the cheekbone, and a very light iridescent apricot on the highest point of the cheekbone. Sweep this lightest luminous blush across the forehead just at the hairline, on the tip of your nose and to round your chin for a further candlelit effect.

AGELESS BEAUTIES

First, you're going to ignore that silly advice that tells mature women to wear just a dab of makeup now that you are "a certain age." A true Ageless Beauty knows that every year it takes one more product to achieve a totally natural look. And you'll use the works.

1 *Moisturizer.* Products with collagen/elastin or cell-renewal elements *do* make a difference, not only in the way your skin looks but also by improving texture and elasticity. Enough said?

2 *Sculpturing.* Even though you may not wish to do an involved sculpturing job on your face, every Ageless Beauty will benefit from two techniques. Shadows and circles under the eyes make you look tired and old, but the standard shadow cover-up that comes in a tube like lipstick is usually much too heavy, settling into a few expression lines and turning them into bona fide wrinkles. Instead, use a creamy translucent highlight. Shop for one that has a peachy overtone, and avoid products that are too stark white.

3 *Foundation.* You need a makeup base that is light enough to slide over any tiny expression line, yet one that has enough coverage to give you a look of ageless vitality. So many liquid makeups seem to go on like a slide of hand lotion and totally disappear. You may need to mix one bottle that's too translucent with a bottle that's too opaque to create the proper mix of light coverage. Beware of makeup bases that are too tan, too pink, or too dark. Dark makeup will make your skin look leathery and accent wrinkles. Choose beige peachy tones to match your skin or one shade *lighter* (this reflects the light and minimizes tiny lines). Do rely on blushers to give your face that flush of healthy youth and color—I've noticed that many mature women get this equation upside down. They attempt to add color to their faces through heavy, too-dark foundation, and then wear almost no blusher at all. This is wrong. The indispensable cosmetic for the mature face is . . .

4 *Blusher.* Translucent is the key word here. Liquids, gels, creams. Any warm color that lets your skin shine through will create a healthy, ageless effect. Avoid any product that has a blue undertone. Choose instead peach, apricot, coral, even bronze. Powder blushes are much too heavy for you, and their matte finish can create a flat, slab-like effect. But blushers applied as I'm going to show you now, in three colors and textures, can give your cheeks the high rounded contours of youth. Hooray!

A. Smile into your mirror and apply cream or gel blush on the high point of your cheek. Pat it into a circle about the size of a half dollar, and use enough color. The highest intensity of color will be on the "apple" of your cheek. Blend the edges of your pastel "half dollars" up, up toward the temple and allow color to set.

B. Next, use a translucent liquid blush to create a wash of solid color over the entire cheek area, possibly on the bridge of your nose, on your forehead at the hairline, and don't forget a dab just under your chin to minimize the tiny pad that may have appeared in the last few years.

C. You can further lift the cheek contour by adding a dot of pearlized highlight (pearl lip gloss is great for this effect) on the very highest point of your apple contour, just as if you were painting the highlight on an apple. Very gently blend the edges of this highlight up and out toward your temple. Can you see how these colors and textures have created a three-dimensional effect that gives the illusion of a lifted rounded contour?

5 *Powder.* What trick do makeup artists use to create the effect of age? Lots and lots of powder, which accents every line and wrinkle! That should explain why I advise a minimum of powder for your ageless face. If your skin has a soft luster or sheen, good! That's the look of youth. Extremely oily skin is usually a problem for young skin. But if your nose does get shiny, use "Face Saver" blotters instead of a powder puff. There is one place that you will be using powder—when you apply your eye makeup. Details coming up in Day 6.

Ageless Beauties with dark brown or black skin may not be using makeup because in the past products were very unsatisfactory. Black is beautiful today, with foundations and blushers designed to overcome the ashen effect that old-fashioned products used to create. Be aware that black skin tends to darken as it ages. Your foundation color may need to change as you get older. Dark, plum-toned blushers are an old-fashioned approach to adding color to dark skin. Choose instead from the wonderful array of copper, amber and bronze tones. Powder—both loose and pressed—should be a fraction of a shade darker than your face as it tends to "lighten" on your skin.

Day 4 — Beauty Essence Workout: Conquer Makeover Sabotage

About this time in many makeovers, an insidious, self-defeating attitude may be lurking in the shadows. I call it makeover sabotage, and today we're going to face it head on! This sabotage usually involves not practicing the beauty techniques outlined in each daily lesson because new ways of thinking, new ways of doing take a little effort. It's much easier to continue to express one's self in the same old way—but look, every skill is a little difficult when we first try it. Think of your first ride on a bicycle! Practice will make each step in your makeover increasingly easy, until the new techniques become old, familiar friends. Further, practice makes it *You!* It feeds into those positive programming techniques of inner dialogue and positive visualization that I described in Days 1 and 2.

What else constitutes makeover sabotage? Skipping a step in the carefully thought-out Close-up program because "I don't want *that* much change." Every step in my Close-up Makeover plan is important—and spelled out in easy stages. This plan has been carefully developed, tried and tested. Your successful Close-up Makeover will bring you the very same inspiring payoffs, both in outer and inner beauty, that other women throughout the country have enjoyed. It works—but only if *you* do. Of course, this doesn't mean adopting a grim, final-examination attitude toward the process. Your makeover is play, so review your P.Q. test and indulge. Don't "take the time"—*give* yourself time to do each beautiful step in your Close-up. You deserve it! And you deserve not only the beautiful Close-up results but the fun of getting there.

Eight

DAY FIVE

The Eyes Have It

On television, when I'm designing a Close-Up Makeover, I always turn the spotlight immediately on a woman's best feature. And that's what you're going to do today.

Women often ask me, "How will I know which is my best feature?" Really, there's no contest at all. Only your eyes can truly be considered for this starring role. Colorful, mobile and expressive, they are the accent points of your face and naturally take center stage. A pert nose, dimpled chin, or perfect complexion can only be considered featured players in the continuing drama of the face.

First, let's have a look at the most common mistakes in eye-makeup application. So many of the women I see, in an attempt to accent their eyes, allow their eye makeup to overwhelm this subtly expressive feature. In effect, their too-obvious eye makeup becomes a raucous scene-stealer. Too-timid eye makeup is just as bad, giving your face a forgettable "don't call us, we'll call you" image. These are the most common eye makeup mistakes:

- Eye shadow color too bright—the NBC peacock would be green, or blue, or purple, with envy

- Eye shadow not blended—again, too obvious an effect
- Eye liner and/or mascara too heavy and obvious

Color mistakes in eye-shadow choices are by far the most common and obtrusive, and the easiest to correct. Blending shadows skillfully and applying eye liners and mascara effectively are also fairly easy when you follow my step-by-step guide. In fact, it all becomes rather easy when you understand the real purpose of eye makeup.

It's easy to see why most women have been misled about eye makeup—the world of fashion has too often taken it into bizarre and garish realms that are terrific on the cover of *Vogue* but pretty weird on *you* as you stride into a meeting at 9:05 A.M.

There's absolutely nothing wrong with a *hint* of color in your eye-shadow palette but only in a quiet, supporting role. The purpose of eye makeup is not to add color to the eye area or turn your gray eyes into royal blue show-stoppers. Instead, it must be just what the name implies—a subtle shadowing of the eye area with these goals:

- To frame the eye
- To "open" the eye, making it look larger; to add contrast to the white of the eye
- To create the most attractive bone structure possible

Your Basic Close-up Eye Makeup Plan

The most flattering, effective eye makeup just continues the basic light and dark contouring techniques you learned in Day 4. You'll use light creams and powders to lift, accent, and bring forward specific areas, and dark creams or powders to shape, minimize, or indent other areas. *Shadow contouring is the most important part of your eye makeup.* If you master contouring, you'll be ready to add accent and emphasis with eye liner and mascara.

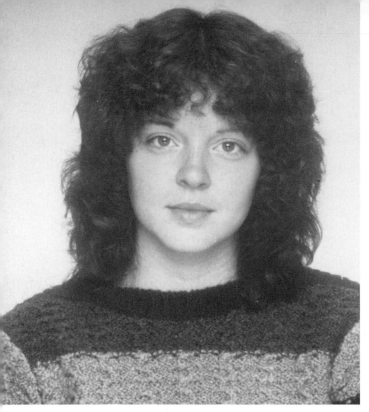
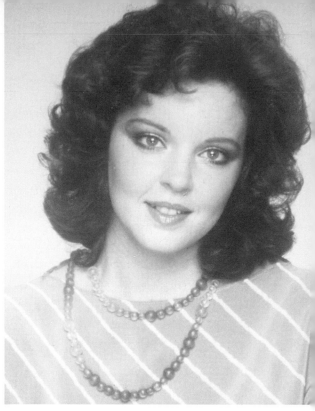

The most flattering eye makeup uses subtly blended shadows.

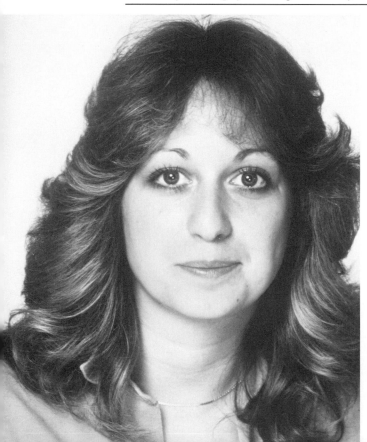
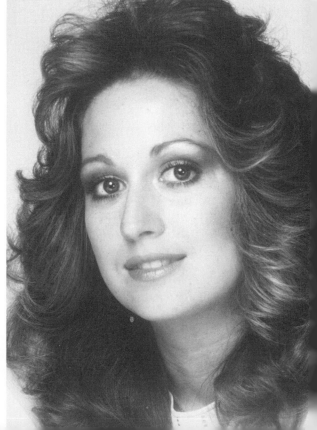

1 Completely cover your eye area with foundation. This very first step is often a surprise to the women I work with in my television make-overs. As you will see, it serves as your base, and is essential to successful eye makeup application.

2 Apply a light-colored cream base over the upper eyelid and into the eye crease. This cream base can be the same cover-up cream that you use for camouflaging under-eye circles. Pat, pat! Blend, blend! If you are using a powdered shadow for dark contouring, you should next powder your eyelids lightly, using translucent face powder or fine baby talc. For fast and easy application, use the Big Daddy powder brush.

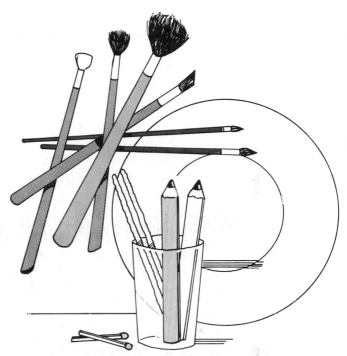

Tools of the trade: Makeup pros use an artist's collection of pencils, brushes, sponges—and some surprising but useful oddities to create unforgettable eyes. Here's my list of basic eye makeup items you can use, depending on the Close-up Portrait you choose to express your beauty temperament:
1. Big Daddy brush: large brush for powder, overall blending
2. The Wedgie: essential for application of powdered eye shadow
3. Sponge-tipped applicator: for applying and blending both powders and creams
4. Fine eye-liner brush
5. Fluff brush: for applying subtle veils of powdered shadow, for color layering
6. Medium eye-liner brush
7. Fatsos: big, soft, eye-shadow pencils
Oddities:
8. White pipe cleaners: terrific for cleaning up smudges, blending small areas
9. White saucer and matches: for soot secret!

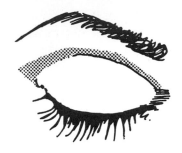

Smooth a band of dark shadow into the eyelid crease.

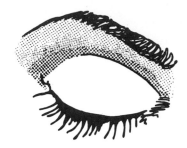

Lift and soften eye contour by blending dark shadow over orbital bone.

3 Smooth a band of dark shadow—brown, gray, mushroom, taupe or some other neutral color—into the eyelid crease. This dark shadow will outline the upper eye socket—in effect, rimming the eyeball itself. To understand what you are trying to accomplish, close your eyes, press your index finger around your upper eye socket. Be aware that the eye is, indeed, a ball covered by the delicate eyelid. Feel the jutting orbital bone that forms your upper eye socket? That's what you'll be contouring with this band of shadow. It should be widest at the outer corner of your eye and it narrows to almost nothing as it sweeps into the inner eye corner. Blend this shadow so that its greatest intensity is at the outer corners and in the eyelid crease. Use your Wedgy brush.

SPOT ANNOUNCEMENT

THIS IS HOW TO APPLY ALL TYPES OF EYE SHADOW EASILY. TO DO YOUR RIGHT EYE, USE LEFT INDEX FINGER TO *GENTLY* HOLD THE RIGHT EYELID CLOSED. NOW YOU CAN WATCH THE AC-TION WITH YOUR RELAXED WIDE-OPEN LEFT EYE AS YOUR RIGHT HAND WORKS. USE THE SAME LEFT-HAND INDEX FINGER TO HOLD YOUR LEFT EYELID CLOSED. THE POINT IS YOU WON'T SQUINT!

4   Blend the dark shadow up, over your orbital bone. This blending technique lifts and softens the eye-socket contour, or creates a hollow where none existed before. The dark shadow should soften in intensity and blend totally away at the eyebrow. Use your Fluff brush for this.

5   Apply eye liner in dark brown or black just above the upper lashes. The liner should continue beyond the upper lashes and into the inner corner of the eye, clearly defining it.

6   Draw a softer line under the lower lashes. This step is a must for all eye types. Are you doing this currently? Try it, you'll adore the way it super-accents your eyes.

7   Apply mascara to upper and lower lashes. Look way down into your hand mirror and brush lashes straight out, not to the side. This movement curls your lashes, and minimizes mascara smudge.

There you have it—a basic eye makeup plan that is fabulously flattering to every eye. I want you to perfect this basic eye-contouring technique *before* you try the more advanced problem-solving procedures that follow.

Eyes Right: Checking for Problems

Your next assignment is to analyze your eyes using the Objectivision techniques we've already discussed. With your newly aware vision, you'll note which of your own eye contours have pleasing proportions and which areas need camouflage and correction.

The following illustrations give you a rundown on how each of these proportions can be dramatically improved. But unless you're already very adept at makeup, don't rush ahead and start your corrections. Just make a check mark beside any contour that matches yours.

First place your Eye-Q Isolation Mask over your hand mirror and study your eyes.

DEEP-SET, HOODED EYES: Contour orbital bone, blend shadows up to eyebrow. Pale shadow extends above lashes, onto eyelids, into deep socket.

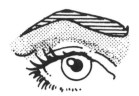 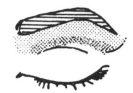

FLAT ORBITAL BONE: Create indentation with dark shadow. Note gradation of color intensity—deepest in eyeball crease.

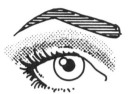 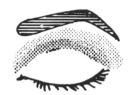

BRIDGE OF NOSE TOO PROMINENT?: Fill in hollows with light shadow.

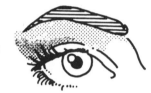 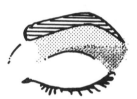

NOSE BRIDGE TOO FLAT?: Create bone structure with shadow.

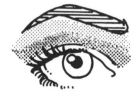 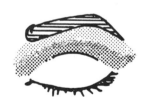

FLESHY EYELIDS: Medium shadow on lid, darker shadow in crease. Use double eye liner—darkest next to lashes, medium intensity above—and lots of mascara.

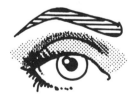 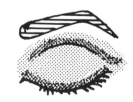

NARROW, DISAPPEARING EYELIDS: Very light shadows on entire eyelids. Eye liner inside upper lashes, below lower lashes. Mascara on upper and lower lashes.

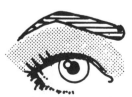 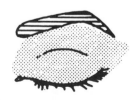

PUFFY, NONELASTIC EYELIDS: Dark foundation makeup on lids, blend to eyebrows. Eye liner inside *upper* eyelid. Mascara.

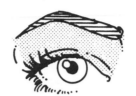 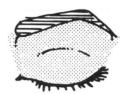

SMALL EYES: Light shadow on eyelid, dark shadow extends beyond outer eye corner, enlarging eyes. Eye liner above upper lashes, below lower lashes. Lots of mascara on top and bottom.

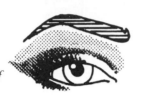 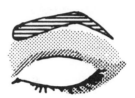

ROUND EYES: Shadow on outer half of lids lengthens eyes. Extend eye liner up and out. Note angular eyebrow shape.

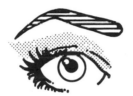 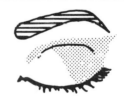

DROOPING, SAD EYES: Dark shadow stops short of drooping outer contour, angles up. Note color intensity at corner. Eye liner stops short of drooping contour at upper lid.

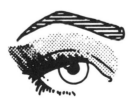 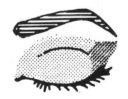

ONE EYE LARGER: To even up eye size, use individual artificial lashes on smaller eye only. Make eye liner wider on smaller eye.

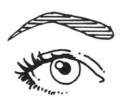 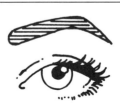

- *The orbital bone (the upper rim of your eye socket).* Is this bone too promi-nent, making your eyes look hooded and tired? Are your eyes too deeply set due to the structure of this bone, making them look smaller or nar-rower than is attractive? Or is this bone flat, leaving your eyes without that shadowed structure that frames them so attractively?

- *The bridge of your nose.* How does it visually relate to the structure of your eyes at the inner corners? Is the nose bridge so prominent that your eyes look too deep by contrast? In other words, do you have two deep hollows at the inner corner of your eyes? Or is the nose bridge too wide, overpowering your eyes and giving your face a heavy, almost coarse appearance? Is the nose bone too flat and without definition—a common problem for Orientals and blacks?

- *Check your eyelids.* Are they too fleshy? A bit crepey? Does your eye structure make your eyelids almost disappear when your eyes are open? Perhaps your eyelids droop at the outer corners? Or are they puffy, either because of age or natural design, filling in the eye crease and making your flattering orbital shadow virtually nonexistent?

- *Analyze the shape of the eye itself.* The ideal eye is large and slightly almond-shaped. How does the shape of your eye compare to that ideal? Is it small in comparison to the rest of your features? Maybe your eyes are *very* round. Do they tilt upward at the corners, or do they dip down?

Now, review your notes from the Objectivision session in Day 1 to see if one eye may be larger than the other. Remember, we learned that this is very common indeed.

Last, your eyebrows complete the picture. We worked on eyebrow placement and shaping in Day 3. If you've been practicing to perfect them, you've made a giant step toward completing the perfect setting for your own two expressive eyes.

I want you to really study the corrections you have checked. Then, gathering your props—pencils and powders and brushes and creams—it's show time! After several rehearsals, you'll be delighted at how quickly you became adept at applying the ultimate flattering eye makeup to your own eyes.

Your Eyes — In Living Color

Before we focus on your individual Close-up Portrait, we must talk about color and how it can be used in real life to add a flattering accent to your eyes. So far, I've discouraged the idea of colored eye makeup. But if you shop anywhere from Neiman-Marcus to Rexall Drug stores, you see a kaleidoscope of colorful eye makeup products—pencils and wands and powders and creams in jars and pots and compacts and tubes—hundreds of luscious colors. These bright eye-catching products are very appealing. Do they have some beautiful place in your Close-up?

Yes, colorful eye makeup plays a bit part—it can enhance your glance but only if it's a soft and subtle tint, a sheer veil of color that does not overpower the delicate color scheme that nature has created in your iris. Now, I'm going to share my three Close-up color secrets with you—secrets that will let you add color to any eye makeup plan easily, elegantly, believably.

Secret #1. Always add a dash of translucent or baby powder to any powdered eye shadow cake. Use a brush (not that little sponge applicator) to blend this talc with the eye shadow. Apply this toned-down shadow to your eyes for a translucent veil of color. If you want a bit more color, blend again with your brush, this time getting more shadow color than talc. Once you start this method, you'll find that you almost never take your eye shadow colors "straight." Compared to the sophisticated pastel created by the above method, almost every product is too garishly bright and brassily obvious.

Secret #2. To change too-bright colors to the misty, airy, shadowy tones that are truly flattering and natural, always mix bright shadow colors like lilac, turquoise or fern with your brown or gray muted basics. For example, bright blue shadow becomes a lovely, misty hint of blue when blended with your basic gray. Again, you'll find that dipping your brush in baby talc will smooth this color mix even more.

Actually, this technique is rather like Renoir painting with eye shadow. The baby powder, like water with water-color paints, dilutes and softens every eye shadow color, helps to mix two or three colors, makes the shadow mixture float onto the eyelid surface. And it will stay and *stay*.

SPOT ANNOUNCEMENT

TO SOFTEN AND SUBDUE LIQUID (WAND) OR CREAM EYE
SHADOW COLORS, BLEND WITH FOUNDATION FOR A MISTY,
FRENCH IMPRESSIONIST EFFECT.

On the other hand, if you want to *intensify* the color of powdered eye
shadow cake—for a dramatic eye liner—moisten the cake and use it just
like water color. This is also effective for tiny, little accents—a lilac line
just under the lower lashes, for example. Or a wide, translucent line of
bronze just above your upper lashes.

Secret #3. A little warm color in the form of powder-diluted blusher
creates a foolproof sunny finish to your eye makeup whether you use
powder or cream shadow. Coral, peach, bronze—almost any of these
shades will be flattering, provided you dilute the color. Use the large
brush that comes with the blusher, dilute the color slightly with talc, then
brush over your entire upper eyelid area.

A final word on colorful eye makeup. Remember that the color
scheme of your *complete* 10-Day Makeover plan will focus everyone's attention on your eyes. Eye makeup is just part of the ensemble. Flattering
enhanced hair color will intensify your eye color. Foundation makeup
and blushers will dramatize your eyes, making the whites appear whiter,
the iris color more intense. That's why eye makeup, as you have just
learned to apply it, can be subtle and still *very* effective.

Eye Makeup Scenarios for Your Individual Close-up Portrait

THE TRULY NATURAL EYE

Your devotion to the natural look goes beyond the aesthetic and so you
have made an almost mystical commitment to expressing your image in

its most unaffected, most essential form. Still, even you who are completely devoted to the "Be Yourself" philosophy may need to accent your eyes a bit, in order to let the Natural Woman shine through. For this reason, I'm giving you two choices in creating your Truly Natural Eye. Let's start with the most ingenuous, noncosmetic effect you can achieve:

1   Use castor oil (that's right!), patted in a thin film on your eyelids. Blot with a tissue to leave the thinnest possible sheen. Next, brush lashes with a mascara brush *lightly* lubricated with castor oil. This gives the lashes a luster and, in my personal experience, it seems to make the lashes grow. Why castor oil? It's a super lubricator, used in many industries because of its oily, yet nongreasy quality. This oil treatment enhances your Truly Natural Beauty look with a softly gleaming finish.

2   Another effect (with another surprise ingredient) is an eye liner that gives subtle emphasis to the natural look. This trick has been ascribed to the first of the great Westmore movie makeup clan, George Westmore, who pioneered the screen makeup techniques that made stars out of actresses. He believed that this "saucer secret" created a soft subtlety unmatched by standard cosmetics.

Take an old saucer or other china object (no plastic) and a wooden kitchen match. Allow the match to flame against the saucer so that it deposits a smudge of soot. Using a fine eye-liner brush, roll the tip of the brush in the soot and line your eyes, both upper and lower lids. Experiment a little. You'll find that you can smudge this line for a very soft effect, or make it quite definite. You'll be surprised at how lasting this natural liner is, and a bonus is that it's nonirritating for those with allergies to eye makeup.

If you're not an absolute purist, you could complete this smudgy eye liner by using mascara—brown tones for fair skins, black for olive or darker skin tones. Cake mascara, an oldie but goodie, seems to appeal to the nature girls among us and this product is still available at variety stores. But it's not just nostalgia that makes me recommend it—cake mascara colors, coats and separates the lashes with the most natural-looking results. Its uncomplicated formula makes it a boon to those with eye-makeup allergies.

Here are two more tips to give you better-than-natural lashes:

- Moisten the mascara cake with milk rather than water. This gives your lashes more body and thickness.
- If you want really *fabulous* lashes, add a pinch of dry powdered milk to the mascara cake. With water-moistened brush, blend and mix the mascara and milk into a thick creamy paste. Brush liberally on lashes. And don't blame me if people think you're wearing false eyelashes!

Special Effects for Evening.   To accent your eyes for evening, use a dark bronze liquid blush as eye, cheek and lip color. After applying moisturizer, dab the bronzer at the center of the upper eyelid and blend up to and over the orbital bone. Complete the look with black mascara and soot eye liner. To get the right shade of bronze, one that would match your skin if you were lightly tanned, you want a shade that will enhance the natural undertones of your skin—ashier bronze if your skin is olive, a pinky-brick tone if you're very fair, coppery if your skin has golden undertones.

THE CASUAL EYE

Your busy, breezy life style leaves you with little time (or inclination) for elaborate eye makeup designs. The following quick and easy eye makeup story is scripted to fit into your schedule perfectly, yet give your eyes an accent and finished look that will be appropriate for the classic, often preppy, clothes you like so well.

As with the other elements in your Close-up Portrait, you must make an initial time commitment to shop for the simple yet essential cosmetic items needed, and practice to learn the technique. If you'll do these two things, you'll find that this eye makeup plan takes only about forty-five seconds to complete!

These are the cosmetic items you'll need:

- Eye shadow pencils (those fat ones with the very soft lead) in two shades—dark and light, for example, bronzey brown and peachy beige. Or smoky gray and pinky silver. Sometimes these pencils come in a two-leaded, color-coordinated style—light shade on one end, dark on the other—that seems especially adapted to your busy schedule.

- Eyebrow pencils in two colors—light brown and very dark brown will be flattering to most women. If your skin tone is very dark or you want a more obvious effect, choose black and brown for your two pencils.
- A mascara wand in brown or black.
- A blusher in a brownish, bronzey tone. Some makeup companies are making contour powders in a light brick shade. These are effective for you and a favorite tool of all makeup artists.
- A *very* good sharpener for your pencils—pay a bit for it because it will make those eye shadow pencils go further. *Tip:* when you want to sharpen those big soft pencils, put them in the freezer for a few minutes, then sharpen. You'll see. They don't break.
- A sponge-tipped application for blending.

Now that you've gathered the equipment, here's your easy-on-the-eyes plan for day and evening.

1 Apply moisturizer and makeup base to entire face, being especially careful to blend foundation makeup onto eyelids. Blend carefully into eye corners.

2 While your makeup base is still a bit moist, take the dark eye-shadow pencil and apply to the eyelid crease and the outer corner of your eye.

3 Use the lighter pencil and draw a band of color below the eyelid crease (that's right, on the eyelid). Work quickly now, and blend the dark-penciled color *up* onto the brow bone, the light-penciled color *down* onto the eyelid. Use your sponge applicator and you'll find that these shadow pencils blend beautifully, especially when applied to makeup-moistened lids.

4 "Set" this shadow with a quick application of bronze, brick-toned blush. Apply the powdered blush on eyelids, then go ahead and brush this blush onto cheeks, forehead, bridge of nose, as you learned on Day 4.

5 Take the darkest eyebrow pencil and line the upper eyelid, right next to the lashes. Does it smudge a little? Good. That's just the soft effect you want. You may also want to put a soft, smudgy line under the lower lashes for a P.M. effect.

6 Apply mascara, using the liquid wand type that brushes and separates the lashes at the same time mascara is being applied.

That's it—don't slam the door on your way out!

Special Effects for Evening. Instead of using powdered blusher to set eyeshadow, use powdered eyeshadow, pastelled with translucent powder, in the color of your choice.

THE CONTEMPORARY EYE

You're the Contemporary Woman and you have it all—because you *do* it all—wife, lover, mother, working woman, you play each role beautifully because you understand that you *can* play several roles.

During business hours, when you wear your Contemporary Face, you project an image that says, "Female I am, fragile and feminine I'm not."

Eye contact is a very powerful element in any human interrelationship. In the contemporary business scene, you can use your eye makeup to give your eyes more power and authority. As you read through this plan, you'll note that, unlike the eyes in the other Close-up Portraits, it's all right, even desirable, to create a hint of hardness in your eyes. Not hard in the sense of cheap, but rather in the true sense of the word—hard, strong, unshakable.

Another consideration for you is to counteract the draining effects of fluorescent light in the work place. Almost every business uses them, and their blue-white color level can make you look tired and enervated at 9:00 A.M.—not the dynamic success image you Contemporary Beauties want to project.

Here's what you'll need to create the authoritative Contemporary Eye:

- Liquid wand eye shadow in a warm brown tone; burgundy, wine, brandy brown. This warm brown shade is suitable for all but the darkest complexions and all eye colors. The idea is to counteract blue-white fluorescents, at the same time encouraging your iris color to stand out. This won't make your blue eyes bluer, but it will make them attention-getting. And brown eyes look darker, larger, compelling.
- Powdered cake shadows for a finishing accent. Putting powdered shadows over the liquid type gives you a finish that lasts all day. Choose another brown shade that contrasts with the liquid shadow you have chosen. Perhaps a more golden brown, or a bronzed tone.
- Black or brown mascara and a dark eye-liner pencil.

Turn on your telephone answering machine, sit down at your efficient makeup table, switch on the lights, and let's get started.

1   Apply eye makeup over your basic makeup—moisturizer, camouflage cream and foundation base. Because fluorescents will magnify any hint of shadows or dark circles under your eyes, carefully apply that camouflage or cover-up cream. Even if you don't think you need this product, use one anyway. For quick and easy application, I recommend a cover-up stick.

2   Apply the cover-up stick directly under your lower lashes allowing the light line of cream to extend up and out at your eye corners, to create an energizing lift. Take the unused sponge applicator from one of your cake shadow compacts and use this to blend the cover-up cream right under the lower lashes, then smooth and blend down onto the area under your eye. Pat, and pat again, with your fingertip.

3   Take the shadow wand and draw a crescent of warm brown color in your eye crease. Blend the color up over the orbital bone and then blend away to nothing on your eyelid.

4   Use the powdered shadow for a finishing accent and to set the shadow contour. Use Secret #1, the talc trick, to dilute the cake color, making it easier to blend. You may wish to add a warm highlight in the form of peach or pink shadow. Fine, but don't use an iridescent type—too glitzy for most business images. Use your fingertip or a sponge applicator to put a peachy highlight on the center of the upper eyelid. That's all. No fancy stuff. No gleamers under the brow bone, no tip-tilted eyes. You mean business.

5 Apply the dark eyeliner in a *narrow* line at the upper eyelashes and just under the lower lashes. Take a Q-Tip and smudge this lower line. You may choose to make your eye liner a bit heavier at the outer eye corners, but this should create just a suggestion of lift. Be sure that this dark eye liner clearly defines the inner corners of your eye, upper and lower. To accomplish this, apply the eye-liner pencil line just inside the eyelashes, on the little rim of skin inside the eye corner. Do the same on the lower lid. The idea is to have your eyes completely, though delicately, rimmed with liner.

6 Finally, apply *one* coat of mascara on your lashes, for definition only. Long, fluttery eyelashes are definitely flirtatious (see The Alluring Eye) so don't accent this feature. I've recommended black or brown mascara and there's a little color switch here. Brown-eyed beauties should experiment with both colors. The black mascara may be too harsh when coupled with that black eyeliner. Blue- or green-eyed types will usually look just fine with the black mascara, black eyeliner. This combination gives your light-colored eyes an authority they need.

Whether your eyes are blue, brown, green or hazel, following this scenario will create eyes that command attention in the contemporary business world, and create the image to consolidate your position. I mean, these are the eyes that give you the confidence to say, "I love you, Roger. But you're fired!"

Special Effects for the Night Scene. Because the Close-up Portrait of the Contemporary Beauty is designed to create an image that builds success in the business world, I really don't see an adaptation of this theme as being effective for evening. That is, unless evening means a business conference or seminar. No, for big evenings or intimate nights, the Contemporary Beauty chooses another portrait to express herself.

Still, there are occasions when the Contemporary Eye needs an added definition and power. If you are making a presentation in a large boardroom, or if you must give a report or chair a meeting in an auditorium, you can increase the emphasis of your eyes by adding more black liner, using black mascara (whatever your eye color), and finally, by using the following little makeup accent from my stage actor's bag of tricks.

At the inner corner of your eye, just inside the black liner, draw a delicate red line, using a lip-liner pencil in true red. You can also make a tiny red dot, just at the point of the inner eye corner. *Careful now.* The idea is to create a tiny red accent that intensifies the eye whites. The red color makes this technique effective from a distance. And, carefully done, it's unnoticeable up close. You can also place a dot of iridescent white right next to the eye corner, between the eye and the bridge of the nose. Use a pearly eye shadow pencil for quick and easy application. This, too, will make your eyes look more defined from a distance, yet does not look bizarre up close.

THE DESIGNING EYE

Eye makeup gives you, the Designing Beauty, an opportunity for the most elaborate yet subtle artistry. As always, you avidly study the fashion magazines and experiment with the design innovations spelled out there, and you'll create some of your own. But while you are aware of all the elements that change from season to season, you do have a basic eye makeup plan geared to flattering what *doesn't* change—the basic structure and color of your eyes.

Fashion, not fad, is your theme. Let's say the beauty editors breathlessly tell you, "The Android Eye is 'in.' Line your eyes first with metallic silver, layer on gold and platinum up to the eyebrows." Unless you're booked for an appearance on "Solid Gold," avoid brash, punky colors, and extreme applications—for example, metallic pink eye shadow, bright blue or green mascara. In other words, follow fashion, but remember it's your *eyes,* not your eye makeup that we want to see.

Whatever fashion's dictates, eye makeup seems to take two paths: the colorful eye—a blending of sometimes surprising colors and textures to create a mini work of art; and the monochromatic eye—variations on a single color theme.

The Monochromatic Eye. The purpose is to glorify, not alter, your very own eye color, so be meticulous in choosing makeup colors that exactly reflect the nuances of your own eye color. Don't merely think in terms of brown eyes, for example. Is your iris hazel? Sherry? Deep brown? Blue eyes can be gray, cool blue, violet-toned, or with a hint of turquoise. Incidentally, if your skin is fair and you have brown or hazel eyes, check out the cosmetic lines designed for dark-skinned beauties. You will find a wealth of color inspiration in these products. This is what you'll need to create the monochromatic eye.

- Powdered shadow in three shades of your chosen color—light, medium and dark
- Two eye-liner pencils—one light, perhaps with a bit of metallic gleam, and one dark
- Mascara with a *subtle* undertone of your chosen color, i.e., midnight blue (for blue eyes), olive brown (for hazel eyes), plum brown (sherry eyes), black brown (deep brown eyes)

Here's the plan.

1 Prime your eye area with foundation.

2 Fill your eye-shadow blending brush with the medium tone eye-shadow powder and apply to eyelids, being sure to completely cover lids from the very inner corner at tear duct to the outer curve. If you've done this correctly, you will have a perfectly delineated eyelid in your theme color.

3 Using the darkest shade of eye shadow, brush a line of color in the crease above the eyelid, starting at the outer corner of the eye and sweeping toward the tear duct. Refill brush with this darkest powder color and apply a wedge of shadow color at the outer eye corner. This wedge-shaped color block will encompass the outer edge of both upper and lower lashes, and will angle up toward the temple.

4 Using the lightest color in the eye-shadow trio, dilute with baby talc and blend this lightest color over the entire eye area, from lashes to eyebrow. This lightest shadow application should "take the edge off" and put your color theme into soft focus.

5 With the darkest eye-liner pencil, use the model's trick of lining the *inside* rim of your upper eyelid. Looking into your hand mirror, put your head back, lift eyelid up with the left hand, and using the sharpened but very soft eye-liner pencil, simply run a line of color on the inner lid directly underneath the lashes. *Do not use pearlized pencil for this purpose.* You will use the lighter, possibly pearlized, eye-liner pencil to draw a line from tear duct to outer corner *above* the upper lashes and to completely line the eye underneath the lower lashes.

6 Complete the monochromatic eye makeup plan with a thorough application of color-coordinated mascara. Note: if this color plan is too subtle and understated for your taste, add a touch of pizazz via a totally unexpected spot of light, bright eye-shadow color applied at the very center of the eyelid and/or directly under the arch of your eyebrow.

The Colorful Eye. The monochromatic eye plan can be revved up for evening with the simple addition of a color wedge of iridescent blusher: pearlescent for blue eyes, gold-gleamed for brown. Take your Big Daddy shading brush and smoothly glide iridescent blush over the entire upper eye area. Sweep color up and out toward the temple. Next, apply iridescent blush to the high points of your cheekbone and angle up to meet the sweep of color at your hairline. The effect will be an almost imperceptible masque of rosy color, lifting all cheek and eye contours and adding sparkle to the whites of your eyes. This will turn the spotlight on your eyes in the dimmest light.

More P.M. Plans. The secret of changing A.M. into P.M. makeup drama involves the addition of metallic accents—gold or silver, according to your eye color. One easy and inexpensive way to turn all eye-shadow powders into evening dress is this: use translucent face powder that has an iridescent finish to "pastel" all of your cake eye shadows. Finish the P.M. plan with eye liner and pencils in gold, silver or color-coordinated iridescence.

THE ALLURING EYE

Attraction is your game, and the following makeup plan proves you an easy winner. Soft, soft color surrounds the ultra-feminine eyes in the Alluring Face. Fluttering, flattering lashes make every glance potent with promise—even if you're thinking about your grocery list.

This is what you'll need:

- Powdered eye-shadow cake in two shades of the same soft color. This is the one time when I recommend obviously colorful eye shadow—with restraint, always restraint. Many cosmetic companies offer eye shadow compacts in twin shades of the same *pastel* color. For example, lilac and violet, sea green and turquoise, or olive green and golden green. (This last is terrific if you have olive or brown skin tones.)
- Cake blush-on in pink or peach.
- For evening, loose powder with iridescent gold or silver gleam.
- Individual artificial eyelashes add an irresistible finish; choose black ones unless you are very fair.

Now, slip into your black lace peignoir, tie your hair back with a pink satin ribbon, and let's get started.

1   As with all eye makeup plans, you'll start with the eye area primed—moisturizer, shadow cover and foundation smoothly applied. Wait a few minutes until foundation is fairly dry.

2   Take your eye-shadow blending brush, dip into baby talc, then brush over the lightest color in your eye-shadow duo. Let's say you're using the violet/lilac combo. With the talc trick, you'll have a muted, very pastel lilac powder that will smoothly glide over your eye area. Brush this powder over the entire upper eye area, covering the orbital bone and softly blending away at the brow line. If you've done this correctly, you'll have a soft wash of color over your entire eye area. Too little color is better than too much. You can always add more. In fact, like Salome, your second veil of color will be a bit more intense. You'll apply it starting at the outer corner of your eye in a soft, wide band right in the eye crease.

3 Next, take an eye-liner brush and, using the lilac color undiluted, draw a band under the lower lashes.

4 Now, you'll add shadow accents with the darker shade, in this case violet. Using your blender brush, again dilute the shadow color with talc, and brush a band of dark diluted color into your eyelid crease, contouring your eyes to enhance your natural bone structure. With a moistened eye-liner brush, use this darker shade as an eye liner, creating a smooth violet line under the lower lashes, a wider line at the upper lashes. Notice that the effect is still one of soft pastel color. Even your eye liner is soft and misty. The idea is, "violet pools a man could drown in."

5 Now, add a touch of warm blush to the center of each eyelid. (You can do this with your little fingertip.) Take your Big Daddy shading brush and dilute this warm blush with talc, then brush over the orbital bone and up to the eyebrow. Shake all the powder off the blending brush and give your entire eyelid area a blending sweep to remove excess powder, to blur and further soften all the colors.

6 Mascara—lots of it—is your one dramatic accent. But comb your lashes carefully to create a softly feathered effect. Individual artificial lashes are an irresistible addition to this look. And believe me, they're so much easier to apply than strip lashes. I have developed my own, unique method for applying these lashes and, with minimal practice, almost anyone can become adept. Here's how.

Choose the lashes that are specifically designed for individual application. I've found that trying to cut up strip lashes into little clumps, as some makeup experts advise, is totally unsatisfactory, frustrating, and leads to some very unladylike language indeed. Also, my method calls for surgical glue (buy it at any drug store) rather than the transparent, *very* permanent eyelash glue that is usually recommended. I personally feel that this glue can be dangerous. If it gets into your eyes or is smeared onto other lashes, it's a disaster! And this permanent glue seems to pull your own lashes right out by the roots when the artificial lashes fall off. On the other hand, surgical glue is nonirritating, no big deal if smeared and smudged where it doesn't belong, and is water-soluble. Yet following my directions, your individual lashes will stay on beautifully for three or four days.

Incidentally, I can't overemphasize the importance of a good magnifying mirror—one that is on a stand and frees your hands for makeup artistry. Now you'll see how invaluable this tool is.

Using tweezers, pull one tuft of individual lashes off the plastic tray. For greater control, tweezers should be quite close to the tied base of the lashes, and not at the feathery tips. Dip the base into surgical glue (I usually put a dab of glue onto the lid of the box that the lashes come in) so that you have only covered the tied base completely. Don't drown that teensy lash in glue, or you'll be a sticky mess. Now, looking down into the mirror, place the little lash onto the top of your upper lid and nestle it into the base of your own lashes. I usually place four or five lashes at the center of my upper eyelid, but you may wish to use them in the outer half of your eye. Here's where individual lashes can be very effective in creating a more pleasing eye shape. Don't forget to review your Eye-Q analysis and place lashes accordingly. Warning: you must wait for these lashes to dry completely. Then brush on a final coat of mascara. *Gently,* please.

If you remove your eye makeup carefully and avoid rubbing the lashes when you are in the shower or washing your hair, they'll stay secure for several days. Certainly, they'll still be on the morning after. . . . I mean, there's no telling where alluring eyes will lead you!

Special Effects for the Evening Eye.   Just intensify your basic colors, using the same basic technique. Line your eyes with the deepest shade of color. Finishing powder with gold or silver flecks will add Emmy-award-winning drama.

THE AGELESS BEAUTY

"Eye Beauty After Forty," the article proclaims, but then goes on to add one limiting idea after another: "little eye shadow, no eye liner, now that you're a certain age, and a subtle touch of mascara, if you're careful." Nonsense! You're a fabulous grown-up woman with wit and wisdom and love and passion to express through those eyes of yours. Forget that timid "sliding into your golden years" stuff, and have gorgeous eyes whatever your age.

The best basic plans for you to follow are the Contemporary Eye, the Designing Eye, or the Alluring Eye. Above all, be sure to wear eye liner. Think about it—the image of the older person is one whose eyes have become faded, almost vague, so forget all that advice about *less* eye makeup, *softer* eye makeup, and so on. You need *everything!* But when you're through, well, *you'll have everything*—experience plus beauty plus confidence. Look out world!

Now, here are some specific tips.

1 Indispensable eye makeup items for you: mascara and eye liner. *Do* wear eye liner—it's essential to avoid that vague look mentioned above. Practice the model's technique of lining your eyes *underneath* the upper eyelashes. Use very dark brown (for brown eyes) or midnight blue (for blue eyes) eye-liner pencil. Be sure the pencil is sharpened to a fine point, then hold the tip between your warm fingertips to soften the lead and make it glide on more smoothly. Use this same eye-liner pencil to draw a dotted, smudgy line among and below the lower eyelashes.

2 If the skin around your eyes is in great shape, apply mascara to upper *and lower* lashes. Remember, mascara is a must for eye beauty. If you seem to have an allergy to liquid mascara, the cake form (an old friend still available at variety stores and theatrical makeup houses) is wearable by almost everyone. Here's one case where a step back in your time machine will pay beauty dividends. For details on super lashes via cake mascara, check out the eye makeup plan for Truly Natural Beauties.

3 If the skin around your eyes is showing its mileage, a bit crepey or wrinkled, here are some further tips.

- Use liquid rather than powdered shadow.
- Apply blending powder sparingly, being sure to blend carefully with Big Daddy blending brush. Powder accents lines, remember?
- Do not use pearlescent or iridescent products except to line upper eyelids.
- That highlight of shiny, pearlized shadow just under your eyebrow is definitely passé. Instead, finish (and set) your liquid eye shadow with a dusting of bronzey-coral cheek blush. This warm blush *over* your eye-shadow base color gives your eyes a vibrant sparkle and makes the whites more brilliant. *Caution:* use your own good taste to choose a blusher that is not too bright. I'm definitely not recommending orange eyelids!

4   What if your eyelids are really a disaster area? Must you forego all pretense of enhancing your eyes with the accompanying lift to looks and morale? Definitely not. Let me pass along a solution that we used in one of my recent television makeovers. The problem: upper eyelids that were so puffy and nonelastic they rested right on top of the upper lashes; the contour was completely engulfed by those crepey puffy lids. Every attempt to add eye shadow just accented this depressing and aging contour. Here is the effective solution that we developed.

A   Instead of eye shadow, use tan foundation makeup three or four shades darker than your overall makeup. Apply this dark foundation over your puffy eyelids from lashes to eyebrows.

B   Be careful to apply this dark makeup in a forty-five-degree angle at the outer eye corner, and let the color fade out close to the eyebrow.

C   Pat and blend this dark foundation with your triangular makeup sponge.

D   Add a finishing touch of eyeliner (remember, bold but muted in color). Smudge the line slightly with a Q-Tip.

E   Mascara on upper and lower lashes completes this camouflage. You'll see. Those crepey, puffy eyelids will magically disappear and you'll look bright-eyed and wonderful.

SPOT ANNOUNCEMENT

USE A MAGNIFYING MIRROR TO HELP YOU WITH YOUR EYE MAKEUP APPLICATION. BUY A STRONG ONE SO YOU CAN REALLY SEE WHAT YOU'RE DOING. NOT SURPRISINGLY, THIS HELPS A LOT. CHOOSE YOUR MAGNIFYING MIRROR WITH YOUR GLASSES *OFF*. AH HA! THAT EXPLAINS WHY THE MIRROR YOU LOVED SO MUCH IN THE STORE, CHOSEN *WITH* YOUR GLASSES ON, IS SO DISAPPOINTING WHEN YOU TRY IT AT HOME, WITHOUT YOUR GLASSES.

Makeup glasses may be just the tool you need to turn you into an eye makeup whiz. These glasses have magnifying lenses which flip down individually, enabling you to work on one eye at a time, while the other eye has the advantage of the magnifying lens.

Day 5 — Beauty Essence Workout: Now Use Those Beautiful Eyes to Express the True You

"They say it all with the eyes." That's director Michael Klinger's description of the hottest movie love scenes on celluloid. But that's hardly news. Everyone knows that "the look of love" is a woman's most potent weapon in the world's oldest game. Yes, your eyes speak volumes, and an easy way to increase their vocabulary is to watch actresses on the screen for a variety of lessons in the technique of eye contact. To make the unspoken messages even clearer, watch your favorite soap opera with the sound turned off. You'll become aware of the multitude of messages conveyed by a look or a studied glance. Eye contact telegraphs interest, assertiveness or allure.

If you're going to make the most of your eyes, you've got to do what actresses do. A little mirror rehearsal will tell you exactly how powerful your eye expressions can be. Stand in front of a mirror and look directly into your own eyes. Smile. And see how that smile creates warmth and emotion in your eyes. Now try to pour all of the warmth and emotion that you can muster directly out through your eyes. Stop smiling but keep that emotional impact pouring out through your eyes. Wow! Powerful stuff! That's your 10,000-volt glance. And I urge you, use it sparingly.

Actually, one of the most seductive of all eye signals is the simplest to achieve. Simply catching someone's eye and holding eye contact longer than usual is a universal message that telegraphs "I think you're interesting and attractive." Surprisingly, a smile dilutes the impact of this message and turns it into a friendly "hello." It's the steady, unsmiling gaze that delivers that KO punch.

Here are other eye movements that invite:

- *The Slow Blink.* Julius Fast, body language expert, points out that the fast blink is interpreted as masculine, but the slow blink is always interpreted as very feminine. Blinking and moving your eyes at the same time is also seductive, says Dr. Henry Brosin of Pittsburgh, Pennsylvania, former president of the American Psychiatric Association. But you don't need a psychiatrist to tell you this is a very seductive eye technique. Try it and see.
- *The Side-long Glance* (a variation of the slow blink). Turn your face to the side and glance out of the corner of your eyes. Blink slowly. Studies indicate that women from the South are more likely to flirt with their eyes in this manner than their Northern sisters. It worked for Scarlett O'Hara and it will work for you.

Now that your eyes are looking their most beautiful, practice these techniques to give your eyes the Look of Love.

The powerful impact of eye language can be used to get you into the boardroom as well as the bedroom. In fact, mixing these messages has detoured many careers. The flirtatious "come on" eye language will no doubt come naturally to you with a little practice, because little girls learn early that charming "feminine" body language gets results. These techniques become second nature.

The assertive body language that is essential for business success must be learned by most women. You'll note that most of the assertive eye language is in direct contrast to the seductive techniques we've just reviewed. As Judy Meyers of the Boston management consulting firm Meyers and Meyers explains, "Eye contact forces a response. It's compelling, and virtually no one is immune to its impact." She also suggests mirror practice. Talk to yourself in the mirror. Practice looking directly into your eyes with a steady gaze. Of course you aren't planning to stare someone down—that's not the idea. Once effective eye contact establishes your concentrated interest, you may glance away. But slide your glance to the side, not down (too feminine), to break that electric contact for a moment. Then bring the eyes back to a level stare.

Remember, eye contact is one of the major signs of dominance in body language. You telegraph uneasiness when you avoid eye contact. If you are talking to more than one person, establish eye contact with each of them as you speak. But you will maintain it frequently and for the longest time with those people who are most important to you or who need to get the full impact of your message.

To study appropriate business expressions, watch the eye language of powerful people who appear on television. "Wall Street Week" is a good source of power moguls and, of course, any powerful or important person being interviewed on the news will be a good role model. Whether for business or pleasure, eye contact establishes and maintains that electric current of concentration. So, here's looking at you, kid!

Nine

DAY SIX

Your Lips

A dialogue without words—key to your emotional temperament—that's what your lips project. Even when you are not speaking, your mouth carries messages to your audience. Mobile, sensitive to your every emotion, you express your image with countless potent movements—the mocking smile that just touches the corners of your mouth, the inviting softness that asks for a kiss, the firm, hard line that telegraphs your displeasure, the tattletale tremor that previews tears.

We have already learned that your eyes are the most important feature in your face, but if your eyes are the stars, your mouth often plays a scene-stealing, co-starring role. As such, it deserves all the attention that its important role deserves.

Lipstick, or lip makeup, to be more precise, has several purposes:
- To accent the delicate and expressive contours of your lips
- To add a healthy color accent to your overall portrait
- To correct and enhance your lip shape
- To protect the delicate skin of your lips

Most women do not know how to accent the beauty of their lips and, in fact, don't have any idea of the creative wonders they can perform with

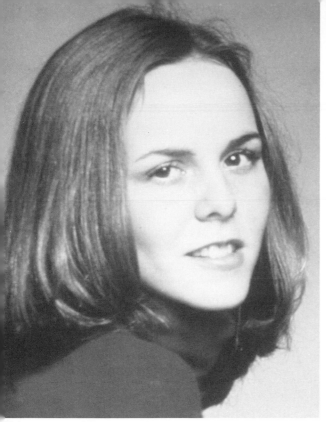
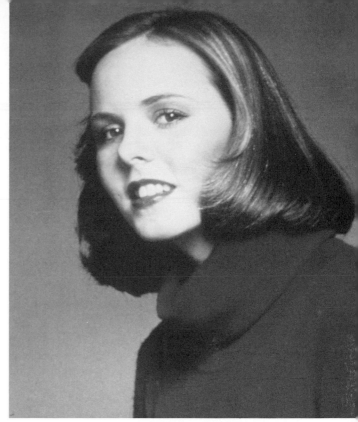

Lipstick enhances the shape of your mouth and adds a color accent to your Close-up.

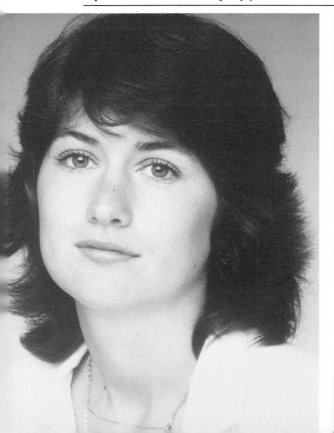
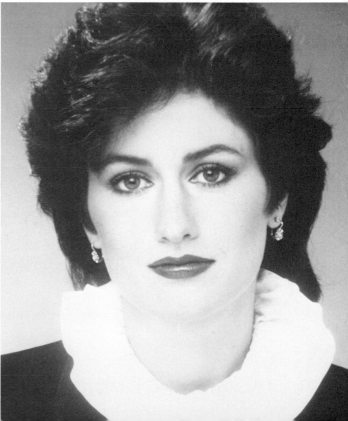

the simple makeup items we have all been familiar with since high school. Do you want a beautiful mouth? You can have it.

Muffed Lip Lines

These are the most common mistakes.

● *No lip makeup at all.* Really, this approach simply doesn't work in today's world. In any urban setting, the lighting, the atmosphere, the mood requires some lip accent. That dab of vaseline, so right in the '60s, makes your face look pallid, out-of-sync with the times, and a bit countrified. Today's woman, whatever her life style, has moved far away from granola and granny dresses and well into the fast-lane tempo of the '80s. So many women work in offices, and under the ever-present fluorescent lights the bloodless look of pallid lips tends to make you look like a zombie. So lip color is essential—even for you Natural Beauties, who often work in offices, too.

● *Out-of-focus, blurred lip lines.* So many women seem to wield that fat tube of lipstick with a hopeful bravado, attempting to create some slight semblance of a lip line but, in the process, masking the true expressive contours of their lips. Using that clumsy oversized lipstick, the routine goes like this: one-two, the upper lip; three, the lower lip; four, slide and smear, rub upper and lower lips to "blend" color. Sure, this is fast and easy—but why bother at all? The slide-smear method simply adds a gash of color to the face, and often makes a woman look messy and overly made-up. Interestingly, the controlled lip makeup guides that I'll be giving you (using every makeup trick) will look much more natural and be much more wearable than the slap-dash approach.

● *Technicolor, not living color.* Common lip color mistakes can dominate and negate the entire color balance of your face, draining color from eyes and complexion. Any shade that is too far from the natural lip color palette will be a jarring note and make your face look harsh and a bit cheap. Avoid shades that are muddy brown, or violent violet, or deep vampire red. But maybe you're one of those women who *wants* to wear Coral Dawn lipstick, only to find that three minutes after application it does a quick dissolve to Midnight Menace Red. If your lipstick seems to be a quick-change artist, I'll teach you to do an easy technique that will keep those shades right on target. Let's start with the most basic lip makeup scenario.

Basic Lip Makeup Plan

Here is the basic plan for lip makeup application. Later we'll discuss the details of color and shape that will suit your own personal Close-up Portrait.

1   Completely cover the lip area with foundation. (Obviously this should be done when applying foundation to eyelids, under chin area, etc.) Remember, we use foundation as the base when creating our Close-up Portrait, just as an artist primes a canvas. So don't miss any facial areas.

2   Use a lip-liner pencil to outline your lips, either following your own lip line exactly or adjusting the outline to create a more pleasing contour. (Details coming up.) For ease and accuracy, choose a pencil with a small lead, and keep the point sharpened.

3   Fill in the outline with lipstick, but do not use that *unwieldy, fat lipstick tube*—you will simply smear the perfect outline you have just created. It's really essential that you use a lipstick brush, liberally filled with lipstick, to stroke the color onto your lips, up to the edge of the lip pencil outline, and—for really professional results—into the lip liner itself. Stroke the lip brush back and forth, blending the lipstick onto your lips. This lip-brush technique is standard procedure with professionals for several reasons. Lipstick stays *on* when brush-blended and the color mellows and develops its most intense shade. And, if you choose not to add lip gloss, lipstick really stays where you put it, minimizing smears on your own face, as well as tell-tale evidence on cups, napkins and his collar.

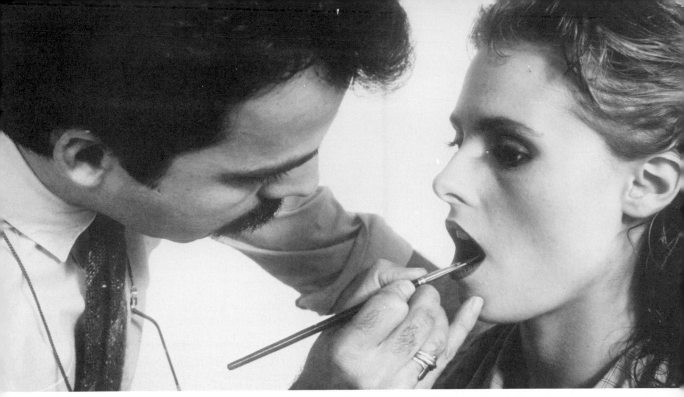

The pros use a lip brush. You should too. Note how the makeup artist steadies his hand with his little finger.

4 Depending on the effect you want, you can either blot lips, setting the lip color even more and creating a slight matte finish. Or, for gleaming allure and the enlarging effects of shine and glimmer, add lip gloss.

That's the basic plan for applying lip color for everyone. Now we'll discuss the many refinements and flourishes that will build your basic lip lines into a major role!

It's Not Just Your Lines, It's How You Deliver 'Em

Now, let's zoom in on that mouth of yours, go over your lip lines, and see what you want to accent and what you want to camouflage.

Step 1. Remove all lipstick and other makeup from your lips and mouth area. Using your Eye-Q isolation mask #4, study your unadorned mouth. Do you like what you see? Is there an ideal mouth, one perfect lip line that you'll want to emulate? While there is an ideal facial shape—oval—and a prototypical eye shape—almond—beautiful lip lines are much more varied, perhaps because our emotional natures are so varied and volatile. Unless you have a perfect Jaclyn Smith mouth, your ideal lip line will probably be the result of careful corrections of less-than-attractive proportions. These are the contours that you'll correct and camouflage:

- *Thin lips.* Full, rounded lips are traditionally and classically beautiful, and thin lips are thought to be less than attractive. All kinds of emotional negatives are associated with thin lips, but if you have them, don't despair. Lots can be done to visually enlarge them (as Cheryl Tiegs and Farrah Fawcett would tell you).

- *Full lips.* Very full, large, "Mrs. Mouth" lips can be too much of a good thing. Sophia Loren and Diana Ross are perfect examples of this problem, beautifully solved.

- *Disproportionate lips.* In some mouths, the upper or lower lip is disproportionately small. Candice Bergen, for example, has a full lower lip with a thin, disappearing upper lip.

- *Out-of-sync lip lines.* These are the common, nonsymmetrical proportions that almost everyone has to deal with. You know, the upper right lip is full, the lower right lip isn't. The upper left lip is thin, the lower left isn't. Do any stars have this problem? Certainly, but we'll never know which ones because this is a problem easily camouflaged.

Using Objectivision, study your mouth to see which of these problems applies to you, then to get an even clearer picture take your lip pencil and draw an outline on the exact edge of your true lip line. This is maybe easier said than done, especially if you have been doing corrective outlining in the past. Be aware that your hands (with their tenacious memory) will try to draw the old correction outline. Concentrate and outline your lips on the exact *natural* line. Now, blot this lip line onto a tissue and study the outline. Can you see where your lip line is not symmetrical? Look at your lips now, and really *see* that outline.

Step 2. Now, you must make some decisions. Which side of your upper lip has the most pleasing proportion? How will you correct the other side to match it up? Do you want to accent your cupid's bow, or soften it? Round it off? Subtly make the high points further apart (to make a broad nose appear more delicate, as Victoria Principal does)?

Look at your lower lip. Is it symmetrical? Probably not. Which side has the most pleasing proportion? How will you make corrections on the less-than-perfect side?

Look at the overall proportions of your lips. Is the upper lip too small, doing a disappearing act, letting your lower lip take center stage? Is your lower lip too full to be pleasing? Or is it small in comparison to the upper? Or are your lips too narrow? Or too full? Decide what you're going to do before you do it!

Step 3. Before you draw your corrected lip line, remove the true outline that you've been analyzing, and pat some foundation over your lips. Using your lip liner pencil, outline the side of your upper lip that is the prettiest. Now, carefully, draw the corrected proportions on the less than perfect side. It may be

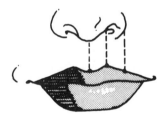

Draw accent points and connect the dots.

helpful to mark your accent points and connect the dots. Use the same technique on your lower lip, outlining the most attractive side, then matching up the other side.

Keep your lips relaxed and smile slightly. Do *not* twist them from side to side, or make an exaggerated "Oh!". You can't possibly follow the outline if your mouth is twisted out of shape, so relax! Always start your lip line at the *outer* corner of your mouth. Do not start at the center and draw the line out to the corner. Why? Because your hand, influenced by gravity, will inevitably create a downward lip line. By starting at the outer corner, you are automatically creating an "up" line as you draw it in toward the cupid's bow. To outline your lower lip, you should also start at the corner.

Step 4. The same contouring principles that apply to facial planes and eyes should be applied to your lips. Yet most women just give lip service to this aspect of their makeup plan. You remember that dark colors and shades make an area look smaller and appear to recede—as in cheekbone contouring. Matte finishes also recede visually. (For example, the large lady in the dark wool flannel suit looks trim.) Light colors and those with a shiny, gleaming finish make an area appear larger and visually bring it forward. (The same lady looks _very_ large in white satin lounging pajamas.) Using these guidelines, here's how to contour lips for camera-ready beauty and more pleasing proportions.

- _Thin lips:_ Use a pink, brick or flesh-colored lip liner. Enlarge lips by drawing lip line just outside your own too-thin lip contour. Accent the fullness of lips rather than the width of them, extending the line over natural lip contour in the center part of your mouth. Next, use pearlized lipstick to apply enlarging shimmer-shine to center of lower lips and in two dots on upper lip.

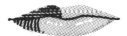 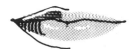 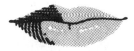

Make thin lips look fuller by extending the lip line just outside lip contour.

- _Full lips:_ Reverse the process described above. Use a darker shade of lip liner. Draw lip line just inside too-full lip contour. Use bright red to deeper red lipstick shades, or coppery bronze tones. To use pink, choose subdued shades, not vivid bright ones. Choose a lipstick with creamy consistency and matte finish—excessive shimmer and shine visually enlarges lips.

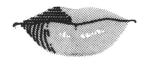 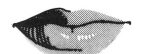 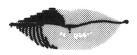

Make full lips more attractive by drawing the lip line just inside your lip contour.

- *Upper lip too full:* Outline upper lip with a medium-dark shade of lip liner. Carry lip liner all the way out to lip corners, accenting width, not fullness, of the lips. Use pink or flesh-colored liner to outline lower lip. Carry the line on the outside of lip line. Fill in both upper and lower lip with light, bright lipstick shade. Using a darker shade, brush over the upper lip, and just inside the lower lip. Blend a bit of the darker shade at lower lip corners.

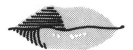 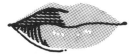 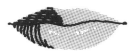

Use dark lip liner on a too-full upper lip to minimize size.

- *Lower lip too full:* Reverse the process just described. Use dark lip liner to outline your lower lip just inside natural contour. Use bright liner on upper lip, drawing the outline just a pencil-line's width outside the lip contour. Fill in upper and lower outlines with medium-bright shade of creamy lipstick. Then use a pearlized lipstick in a related shade, and brush onto upper lip. The light-catching accent makes small upper lip look fuller.

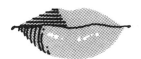 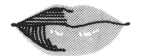 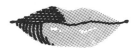

Use dark lip liner on a too-full lower lip to minimize size.

Lipstick color can also be used to enhance your smile, making your teeth look brighter and whiter. Teeth come in a variety of natural shades, and some are naturally more yellow in tone. And cigarettes, coffee and tea can dim the whitest smile. Lipstick shades in bright, true red will make teeth appear whiter. Yellow-toned lipsticks will accent the yellow tones in your teeth. Even a shade or two away from the yellow tones can make a big difference in the brightness of your smile, so experiment a bit. (And don't forget that a good tooth-brightening paste will enhance your Close-ups even more.)

Rehearse Your Lip Lines

I've talked about the importance of carefully and precisely lining your lips to create the most perfect lip silhouette. At this point most beauty books and articles blithely trip along their way, going on to other subjects, leaving you clutching that lip-liner pencil and trying to translate the details of the lesson onto that relatively tiny, soft and mobile canvas that is your mouth. Unless you are very experienced at makeup application, you probably need some guidance in developing the manual dexterity to use your lip-liner pencil effectively. So, let's go back to square one, where you are clutching that pencil with pale-knuckled intensity.

Stress and tension will not create the beautiful and alluring lip line that will complete your Close-up. So, this is essential—hold your lip-liner pencil in the relaxed and confident manner that you would use to write a love letter. Practice drawing the lip line that is most effective for you, remembering to start at the outer corners of the mouth and to sweep in toward the center to complete the cupid's bow. Remember that your lip-liner pencil, unlike a lead pencil, is made of a soft material, so *use a light hand*.

The importance of practicing your new lip line will become very obvious—it's hard for your hand to follow the new directions. Another important point here is to steady or support the elbow of your "drawing" hand. Rest the elbow on the dressing table or (if you're standing at the bathroom mirror) support it with your other hand. Steady the pencil-wielding hand even more by resting your little finger on your chin as you draw. Use this same steadying technique when you use your lip brush to fill in the outline and to brush and smooth the lipstick onto your lips to create a lasting impression. I will remind you again that it's very important to re-educate your hands to produce a new makeup design. If you do not rehearse and practice your new lip line, your hand and that friendly old lipstick tube will produce a rerun of the same lip line that you've been wearing for years.

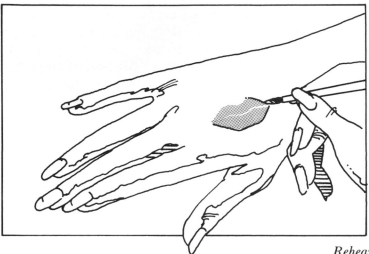

Rehearse your new lip lines.

Close-up Color Secret 1

To prevent your lipstick from doing a quick-change artist number—you know, switching right before your very eyes from true-love red to brazen purple—you need a lip color stabilizer. Believe it or not, these stabilizers come in green or yellow and they keep your lipstick from turning dark. Many of the large cosmetic companies have these bases in their repertoire—you've probably seen them and wondered who in the world would wear a green or yellow lipstick. Now you know it could very possibly be you. Applying an undercoat of green or yellow and then applying your bright coral or true-red lipstick over it will keep your lipstick from turning into an off-color story.

Close-up Color Secret 2

Here is another way of keeping lip color from turning too dark or from being too intense. Remember the technique we learned for softening and subduing harsh eye shadow shades? We can use a similar technique with lipstick shades that, once applied to your lips, turn into Andy Warhol pop art red. Soften and subdue this harsh color effect by using your lipstick brush to blend a dab of liquid foundation with your lipstick color. Apply this softened color to your lips and you'll find that, instead of pop-art shock, you'll have a misty French impressionist effect that will make your lips an appealing work of art.

SPOT ANNOUNCEMENT

YOU HAVE FOLLOWED ALL DIRECTIONS TO CAREFULLY OUT-LINE YOUR LIPS USING THE LIP PENCIL AND THE LIP BRUSH AND YOU STILL FIND THE OUTLINE FUZZY, INDISTINCT AND OUT OF FOCUS. STAND BY FOR THE SOLUTION TO YOUR PROBLEM: PEACH FUZZ ON YOUR UPPER LIP OR—HORRORS!—EVEN A MOUSTACHE WILL DESTROY THE MOST CAREFULLY EXECUTED LIP LINE. IT'S ESSENTIAL TO "CLEAN UP YOUR ACT" AND THERE ARE SEVERAL WAYS TO DO IT. IN THE CASE OF REALLY OBVIOUS AND BRISTLY WHISKERS, ELECTROLYSIS CAN BE A SOLUTION— EXPENSIVE AND PAINFUL, BUT A PERMANENT SOLUTION. AN EASIER WAY AND ONE THAT YOU CAN TRY IMMEDIATELY IS FACIAL WAX. YOU'LL FIND THAT IT'S EASY TO USE AND ALMOST COMPLETELY PAINLESS. YOU DO FEEL A TWINGE WHEN YOU PULL IT OFF—*ZIP!*—BUT BE BRAVE AND READY TO SMILE WITH A SMOOTH, TOTALLY FEMININE FACE AS YOU PROJECT INTO THE LENS FOR YOUR CLOSE-UP. YOU CAN KEEP SMILING TOO BECAUSE THIS WAX METHOD REMOVES THE HAIR ROOT AND SO MINIMIZES REGROWTH.

Lip Makeup Scenarios for Your Individual Close-up Portrait

THE TRULY NATURAL MOUTH

Truly Natural Beauties seem to reject the very concept of lip makeup with all the vehemence and conviction of a television preacher exhorting against sin. But come on, TNBs, a little lip color will add harmony and balance to your truly natural color scheme. There are three approaches to creating the truly natural mouth.

1 Use a lip brush to apply the same bronzing powder you used on your cheeks as a lip color. Use a fine sable lip brush to mix powder and clear lip gloss. Apply this mixture along the true natural outline of your lips. You will find that this has a staining effect which adds color to your lips in a delightfully natural way.

2 You may follow the bronzing application from a dab of lip gloss. For a beautiful finish, use colored lip gloss. Golden or bronze shades create a gorgeous supernatural effect. Also, a touch of this bronzed lip gloss patted onto the high point of your cheekbones will give your face a gleaming sun-goddess look.

3 A variation on the above technique is to outline your lips with an auburn brown or flesh-colored lip pencil (an auburn eyebrow pencil is terrific for this). I hesitate to suggest that you correct your lip line beyond its natural contours, knowing how devoted you Natural Beauties are to the real and true, but if you do cheat a little bit I'll never tell. Then, fill in this more definite outline with bronzing gel. Or, use a liquid lip gloss. The wand-type glosses are available in countless light, natural shades that will give your lips a subtle kiss-of-color that is *au naturel,* yet flattering.

THE CASUAL MOUTH

If I tell you to use a lip pencil, do you think you can do it? Try! It really doesn't involve extra time or trouble. And, in fact, the lip makeup method that I'll be showing you will truly last all day, which is good news for you with your busy schedules. Also, this pencil technique will give your makeup the finished, polished look that is often absent in the Casual Beauty's image. Unfortunately, a messy lip line is too often evident in the portrait of the Casual Beauty. There is a better way, one that you will love because by investing the time in initial lipstick application you will find that your lipstick lasts all day. And a bonus! You will have the polished

American-elegance image that is so perfect for your physical and psychological type.

1 Outline your lips with a lip-liner pencil. Instead of the earth tones that the Natural Beauty chooses, you will find that a lighter, brighter color is more compatible with the sporty, preppy clothes that you wear—true red, bright pink or coral will be flattering to you physically and compatible with your lifestyle. Line your lips carefully following the directions given previously.

2 Fill in the outline. But instead of using that familiar lipstick tube, which is unwieldy and responsible for the smeared, uneven lip lines that one so often sees on Casual Beauties, I urge you to use lipstick in a different, very convenient form. Use a lipstick pencil. These are available in all cosmetic brands and are simply lipstick in pencil form. They differ from the small-lead lip-liner pencil in diameter and in the texture of the lip color itself. Lip liners are much harder and will hold the line better than an LA Rams halfback. But lipstick pencils contain lipstick and so have a softer consistency, and the color is longer lasting than creamy lipsticks because the pencils have a much lower moisture content. Also, for you CBs, the obvious advantages are that a lip pencil is quick and easy to use and does not turn into a gooey mess if left in the sun in your Gucci tennis bag.

3 You can add sculptured highlights to your lips if you choose a pencil that has two colors, a light shade on one end and a brighter, deeper color on the other. These duos are very common. It's simply a question of choosing the one that will do the trick. But again, the point for you busy beauties is the convenience factor—one lipstick pencil does it all.

4 Finish off your lipstick application with a protective coating of sunscreen lip gloss. This will have two effects. The lip gloss will give a natural flattering gleam to your lips, it will protect your lips from the sun, especially important for you who are outdoors a great deal. The advantage of applying it as an after-coating is that during the day (as you dash from one appointment to another) you can reapply the lip gloss, but you won't have to apply your lipstick half as often as you do with the tube variety.

THE CONTEMPORARY MOUTH

When the Contemporary Beauty talks, people listen. That's why it's so essential for you to have a finished-looking, *lasting* lip-line plan that will carry you through morning meetings, a business lunch, and an afternoon conference without requiring major repairs.

1   The first step in this long-range plan is to choose a lipstick that has a long-lasting formula. Almost all cosmetic lines have a variety of lipstick formulas, from translucent lip gloss types to super-creamy, super-mois-turized textures to a long-lasting lipstick that has a staining quality. A simple test will reveal the long-lasting types. Simply stroke the lipstick tube across the back of your hand. Wait a moment, then tissue it off. Long-lasting lipsticks will leave a stain of color, super-creamies disappear completely.

Choose a lip-liner pencil in a close shade. Colors that are best for combating fluorescent fadeout will be bright true red to orange-red to coral shades. Avoid any red tones that carry a blue note.

2   First line your lips following directions given previously. Be sure that your lip-liner pencil has been sharpened to assure a fine, precise outline.

3   Fill in the lip color using your lipstick brush, liberally filled with lipstick. Now, here's the secret to long-lasting color. Brush and brush and brush again, working the lipstick color onto your lips, being careful not to go outside the perfect outline you have drawn. Brushing sets the lip color, and also develops it to its greatest intensity.

4   Blot your lips to remove the excess lipstick. Look at the effect and, if you think it's necessary, reapply a second brushed-on coat of lip color, being careful, obviously, to keep that outline intact. The effect should be a slightly creamy non-matte look, but it avoids the glossy, super-alluring, "kiss-me-quick-baby" image that is so dear to the Alluring Beauty. Re-member, this is the business mouth that talks about contracts, not propo-sitions. (But after hours, consider adding some allure. I mean, all work and no play . . .)

THE ALLURING MOUTH

Let's say it. Mouths are sexy. And lips are for kissing. No one knows this better than the Alluring Beauty and you have a variety of clever plans to call attention to your sexy kissable mouth—without saying a word!

The Alluring Beauty takes what might be called the "Dynasty" approach to creating luscious lips. The two stars of that long-running soap demonstrate two perfect extremes in sex appeal. Scheme One is the softly appealing mouth that makes Krystle so irresistible. Scheme Two could be termed the Alexis look, and who is better at scheming than that gorgeous brunette we love to hate. But, blonde or brunette, choose either of these approaches depending on your emotional temperament.

Scheme One: Krystle

1 Your choice of lip liner is very important. Choose one that is a soft flesh tone, a combination of pink and brown that creates a subtle true-to-life line. Remember that full lips are sexy, so if you have a choice between your natural lip line and exaggerating just a bit, do so—make your lips as full as you can and still keep them looking softly vulnerable and natural.

2 Fill in the outline with a translucent lipstick in pink or coral. This should have more color intensity than the Truly Natural Beauty would choose, but be very close to natural tones. Avoid earthy browns, vivid pinks, bright reds. Run a lip brush over your lipstick to coat it generously with color, then brush onto your lips. Using your pinkie, pat lightly around the edges. You don't want any hard lines.

3 Now for the sensuous surprise touch of lip gloss, applied in a new way that will give your lips a passionate flush of color. Open your lips slightly, and using a lip gloss wand in a shade deeper than your lipstick color, apply a band of color just inside the contour of your lower lip, allowing the color to blend out slightly. At the center of your mouth, bring a line of lip gloss from just inside your lower lip down all the way through the lower lip contour. This gives your mouth a sensuous, pouty look that is still very innocent.

Scheme Two: Alexis

1 For a more intense I-love-being-bad effect, use this plan. The lip liner and lipstick shade that you use will be red, no doubt about it. Remember that in the psychology of color, red is the shade of passion, so don't use any shy pinks or intellectual browns or wine shades. Line your lips with the lip-liner pencil, creating the most curvaceous outline possible, given the natural contours of your mouth. Cupid's bows are sexy, and accenting those two high points will give your mouth that much more impact.

2 Fill in the outline with lipstick. Now, to sculpture even more curves into your lips, use a gold or bronze super-pearlized lipstick and place four highlight dots—two on the lower lip, two on the upper lip (just under the cupid's bow). See how your lips look fuller and more shapely with these highlight accents?

3 Lip gloss supplies the final "come over here and sit by me" moist look that will leave him begging for mercy. But remember, you want your lips to look inviting, not wet and sloppy. Apply gloss in the center of your mouth only, covering the highlight areas.

THE DESIGNING MOUTH

Your intuitive awareness of the total fashion picture makes you sensitive to the delicate nuances of shape and color that create the fashionable mouth. For example, in one season lips may be shaped into voluptuous curves with rounded cupid's bow. In another, the favored lip shape may be a more delicate proportion with fine-pointed cupid's bow. And, in the world of fashion, eyes and mouth trade off the starring role in the face. One season, luscious, brightly-colored mouths take center stage while the eyes play a supporting role. The next season, dramatic eye makeup spotlights the eyes, and mouths are subdued understudies.

The other Close-up Beauties just give lip service to these intricate fashion messages, preferring instead to adapt the high-fashion look with an expression of their own emotional makeup. But you, the Designing

Beauty with your artist's eye and your creative urge to become an expression of the continuing art form that is fashion, will perfect each new trend in color and shape. I won't bore you with the details of lipstick application. You have already perfected the use of a carefully sharpened lip liner, an artist's long-handled flat brush (purchased at your local art store) for a lip brush, the outlining of your mouth (using another artist's 00 brush) with a teensy line of foundation, to accent lips and to camouflage corrections. You clever things know these tricks already. What's more, you've no doubt checked out all the other scenarios in my Close-up gallery and tried on each plan, just for the creative fun of it. So let's get right to some specific plans for designing lips in the '80s. If you look into the face of fashion you'll see that fashion focuses on the mouth. Lips are shaped in the fullest curves possible. Cupid's bows are defined but not sharply pointed.

Here are some color scenarios from the current crop of fashionable faces staring out of the glossy pages of *Vogue, Harper's, "W"*. . . .

● *The Pink Mouth.* Outline your lips with a bright pink lip-liner pencil. Make this outline a bit wider than usual, using it almost like a lip*stick* pencil to give yourself a good, definitive outline. Next, take a wand of liquid lip gloss in a related bright pink, and dab gloss liberally in the center of your mouth. With a lip brush, smooth the gloss to the edges of your penciled outline and blend it into that outline so there's no line of demarcation. (And since you're a semi-pro at makeup, I don't even have to mention to you that using a brush here is essential. Do not try to fill in your outline with that gooey wand tip.) That's it. Pink pizazz!

● *The Very Berry Mouth.* Choose a lipstick in a matte finish, long-lasting formula in a shade from brown-berry to wine-berry. Instead of a lip-liner pencil, use your lip brush to paint your lip line and then fill in entire lip contour with matte berry-toned lipstick. Let color "set" for a moment and then blot. You'll have a soft, berry-stained mouth with no defined lip outline. Now, for the frosting! Using your pinkie, dab a highlight of mauve, iridescent powder (could be eye shadow) on the four highlight contours of your lips—below each cupid's bow and at the center of your lower lip. (Black Beauties will find this look fabulous!)

● *Red, Red Lips.* Yeah! Color schemes for the clothing in the '80s feature so many strong black and neon color combinations that the *very* red mouth is a perfect, even necessary, accessory to keep your face from being upstaged by your clothes. Choose a trio of true-red shades for your lip liner, lipstick and lip gloss. This might be the lineup: lip liner in carmen red, lipstick in true fire-engine red, lip gloss in poppy red—perhaps with a glitz of golden glints. Apply lip liner, lipstick and lip gloss as previously directed. The tone-on-tone red color scheme will give you an attention-getting four-alarm mouth! Seductive and sensational.

THE AGELESS MOUTH

As always, the Ageless Beauty accepts few limitations in creating her most effective Close-up Portrait. Still there are some lip color effects that you should avoid. They will get bad reviews for everyone, but are especially unflattering for the Ageless Beauty: opaque or matte finished lipstick is very 1950s and to be avoided; chalky, too-pastel shades are also relics of those old Doris Day movies; any lipstick that has a blue undertone will make you look older; indistinct out-of-focus lip lines are definitely aging; and of course small, pinched, narrow lips will relegate you to Edith Bunker roles faster than you can say "Stifle yourself!"

As the Ageless Beauty, you have some special problems in applying your lipstick effectively, and I'll be giving you some detailed advice. But first let's talk about the overall effect that you are looking for. Lipstick plans for the Alluring Beauty, the Contemporary Beauty or the Designing Beauty will be most effective for you, so choose depending on your temperament. The lipstick plans for the Truly Natural Beauty and the Casual Beauty do not have enough impact to give you the pizazz that adds up to ageless allure.

Here's a little test to let you find out just how ageless you are. If the Truly Natural Beauty plan has great appeal for you, you are probably stuck in a time warp. It's time to beam up out of the '60s and into the '80s—you're a grown-up lady now, not a '60s hippie, so the natural look that once seemed so right is simply not going to work for you now.

If the Casual Beauty plan has great appeal for you, beware. One of the surest signs of age (not agelessness) is when comfort takes precedence over beauty. If the casual look appeals to you because it's so *easy* to do, remember that as an Ageless Beauty you need more impact and emphasis than the casual look will give you. If the I-don't-have-time element in the Casual Beauty's plan appeals to you, remember that you want to turn *this* time into *your prime time.* You've earned it. It's your turn. So invest the extra time in creating a dynamic ageless portrait for yourself.

Whether you choose the Alluring, Contemporary or Designing Beauty plan to express your ageless portrait, you may find that you are dealing with two age-related problems that seem to prevent the perfect lip line.

First, let's talk about whistle marks. Almost every woman gets them eventually, and it's a black day when your mirror shows you an upper lip that is developing an alarming series of gathers, pleats and wrinkles— aging lines that radiate out from your mouth onto your upper lip, as if your lips were pursed for whistling. One of the most annoying things about them is the terrible effect they have on your lipstick, causing the most meticulously applied lip line to smudge and spread out into those spidery lines on the upper lip. Awful! Well, I have made a wonderful discovery that seems to correct this problem. It's painless, inexpensive, and it works to keep your lip line intact. In addition, it visually re-creates what plastic surgeons call "the white line," that little muscle ridge that outlines and enhances youthful lips but seems to disappear as the years go by.

1   Use an eye-shadow pencil with the smallest lead possible in a light beige or peachy color—this is your "white-line pencil." Apply foundation over your lips, then take your white-line pencil and outline your lips just *outside* the pink portion of your lip line—in other words, just on the outer edge of your natural lip line. If you will be correcting your natural lip line, making it fuller, prettier, or more symmetrical, draw the white-line pencil as close to that corrected outline as possible.

2   With a brownish, tawny lip-liner pencil, outline your lips, making corrections, just inside your "white line."

3   Now, *carefully,* pat a thin, almost-transparent covering of foundation makeup over your double lip line. This is where the professional touch of a makeup sponge is invaluable. When foundation makeup is thoroughly dry, powder over your double lip line. When powdering, you can be sure that the powder won't settle into your whistle marks if you stretch your upper lip down over your teeth. Make a monkey face!

4   Finally, fill in your lips with your favorite lip color, using a lip brush. *Practice.* A lip brush is *the* way to give a perfect finish to this technique. Blot your lips. And see how the "white line" holds lipstick in check, makes lips look younger!

5   Avoid lip gloss. The gleamy, shimmery wet look that is so fashionable is one effect you will have to forego if you have whistle marks.

Besides whistle marks, what else makes the lips of an otherwise Ageless Beauty look old, dated, less than appealing? Almost always, I find that the lip line of potential Ageless Beauties is a distortion of their own true lip shape. A mature woman takes a lip pencil (or lipstick) and, even after completing a makeup lesson, will draw a mouth shape that adds ten years to her face—smoosh!—like that! What's the cause of this distortion? She has programmed her hands to create a dated lip shape, one that through years of unconscious application, has become distorted into a caricature. The answer? Carefully review the section on lip-line analysis. Learn to see what your mouth shape is really like. Then, rehearse! Practice! Consciously train your hands to obey your eye/mind direction in re-creating your own most flattering lip line.

Working with mature makeovers, I find that almost without exception, her true lip line, with a few subtle corrections, is flattering and youthful. So practice getting in touch with your true lip image—a fresh vision, unlocked from that twenty-year mask that you've been painting on. Your mouth will look prettier, younger and, what's more, you'll come face to face with a more vulnerable, more emotional You. Try it. You'll see that form releases feeling!

Day 6—Beauty Essence Workout: How to Project Star Quality for an Impact Beyond Words

In the last few days, you have learned to visually enhance your most expressive features—your eyes and your lips. And you learned some of the effective, nonverbal means of communicating *volumes* through the knowledgeable use of eye contact and the language of the eyes. If you've found that my Close-up eye-contact techniques are dynamite in increasing your personal effectiveness, just wait until you perfect today's lesson. You're going to learn how to project dynamic magnetism—the star quality that adds an irresistible dimension to your Close-up image. The adjective that comes to mind is charisma. Do you want it? You can have it.

This technique of projection, used throughout the centuries in the theater, is a means of dynamically expressing personality in terms of warmth, emotion, energy, life force. Through it we can not only beam out our own personality force, but also become a channel for a greater force of magnetic energy which comes from outside ourselves. Projecting could be called "tapping into the Source," and it's a way of turning up the volume of your personality power. I know that this "tapping into the Source" is a very common technique for all performers. Certainly, it has helped me to be more effective in every step of my career.

How does it work? You consciously project personality power through your "heart center," that sensitive spot in the center of your chest that responds to great emotion. You've had many experiences of projecting from this heart center already—moments of emotion when you've felt a surge of warmth, or compassion, or love or vitality. Think about it. Haven't you felt a charge of energy in your heart center when an experience has touched your heart? Has your heart leapt with joy? And in moments of compassion, haven't you said, "My heart goes out to you"?

In a recent Dick Cavett interview, Laurence Olivier was talking about the heart center and projection when he explained, "I won't do stage work again. I don't have what it takes anymore (gesturing in a circle at chest level, in other words, indicating his heart center). It's something that happens here—a vitality, an extra energy." Theoretically, this energy is always available for us to tap into. Olivier's long struggle with ill health may explain why he no longer feels able to act as a transmitter for this dynamic power. But the point is, *you* can. Here's how.

1   Think of your heart center as a microphone, through which you are going to project any *positive* emotion you choose—warmth, interest, love, compassion, confidence. Now, imagine that you are projecting this emotion toward your audience as if it were a chord of music, surrounding and enveloping them. Breathe slowly and think of this power as flowing *through* you and outward. It is very important to be aware that this is not your *ego* power at work, but rather something beyond your self. Caruso, the sublime tenor, used a variation of this technique when performing and was heard to mutter to himself, just before going on stage, "Step aside, step aside." He explained to a biographer that he was speaking to his own ego. Just practice this little technique in your head. You will soon find that you are projecting this power without having to consciously imagine the golden chord. The same thing will happen with the following technique.

2   Instead of a chord of music, think of projecting a golden beam of light from your heart center. Imagine that it envelopes the person, group or audience that you wish to reach. In order to increase your awareness that this power comes from outside and blends with the light of your own personality, you may wish to think of this as sunlight, flowing through you.

Does this work? Absolutely. Here are just two of the hundreds of success stories I could share with you.

> Last night I went to the first singles party I've attended since my divorce. I felt so unsure of myself—scared to death, really—but before I entered the room, I concentrated on projecting a golden light, as you taught in that seminar, through me and out over the entire room. What happened? First, I felt calm and sure—maybe because I had started thinking of some positive action, rather than negative re-action, you know? And then, well . . . just everyone seemed to want to meet me. It was as if I had become sort of magnetic, in the truest sense of the word. Projection? It works!
>
> (J. K., Denver)

I recently had to give a presentation to several important executives in my company. Even though there were only six people in my "audience," I was understandably nervous—a promotion was riding on the success of my performance. Well, just before I stood up I took a deep breath and mentally projected a chord of music—ta da!—through my heart-center microphone. Then, as I spoke, I remained aware on some level of my consciousness of projecting my thoughts, my ideas, my *self*, out from the heart center on a chord of music. I could feel the power of my personality increase as I did this. I was really "in charge" and impressed hell out of the board. I got my promotion—and an invaluable lesson in success techniques. (M. L. S., Detroit)

I urge you to practice this technique as often as you can to develop your dynamic magnetism. The cab driver, the grocery checker, the tired and bored middle-aged saleswoman at Macy's, the doorman—there are countless opportunities every day to "tap into the Source" and project your personality. What? This sounds phony and too theatrical? Not really. Think about it. What you'll be doing is broadcasting powerful, positive, golden vibes to everyone who crosses your path. And they'll feel it and respond to you in the most positive way. You'll see. Incidentally, you don't have to believe in any mystical aspect of this idea to make it work. Practice, and find yourself becoming that extraordinary woman who is not only physically attractive, but dynamically magnetic. Charisma? You've got it!

Ten

DAY SEVEN

Your Hairstyle: The Mane Event

You probably drew a big red circle around today's date on your calendar because the day you have your Close-up hairstyle is an important one.

You've arrived at today's destination, the styling chair of your chosen hairstyling artist, through a series of careful, deliberate steps. You've been a careful shopper; after all, that's only sensible when you purchase anything. You have with you the results of your homework—your clip file with pictures of hairstyles that you like (and perhaps some that you don't like) and you have your notes. This material is going to help you communicate with your stylist, the first essential step in getting the look you're seeking. We're going to talk more about how to understand the salon terms he may use. But first, let's talk about another means of communication, one that is going to help your stylist envision the look that will complete your Close-up Portrait.

The manner in which you conduct yourself in the consultation gives the stylist a wealth of information about you. Not only the way you look but the impression you make can greatly affect the relationship you develop, for better or worse. By now you have become quite an expert on *you* so handle yourself with energy and self-confidence. The woman who arrives with well-thought-out ideas and specific suggestions but who is not inflexible and who respects the expertise of the staff is seen as a savvy salon customer. Salon professionals would far prefer to work with a woman who knows what she wants than to be faced with one who plops herself in the chair and says "Do me." As Louis Licari says: "One lady will come in and say, 'Louis, I've read all about you. Do whatever you want.' Of course that's a fatal mistake. Hopefully I will give her something that's appropriate because I have faith in my work, but the client should have some control." Now is the time to open that clip file and share with the stylist the Close-up concepts that you have been mulling over since Day 2. Remember, you're not only going to tell the stylist what you want, but you're also going to share with her or him the things that you absolutely do not like—a very important detail.

Once you have explained your goals as accurately as possible, it's the stylist's turn. Sit back and *listen*. This may sound like an obvious bit of advice, but I give it to you after being present at many, many consultations where a woman consults a beauty professional for advice and then proceeds to carry on a one-way dialogue of "I think," "I want," "I know." So remember, you have carefully chosen this professional, and you are paying for his or her expertise (there are no bargain basements in the hairstyling world!). Now is the time to get your money's worth. So I repeat, sit back and listen. If the stylist thinks that your hair is too fine/thick/curly/straight for the style you are requesting, be prepared to revise your notions a bit. Chances are you will be able to get pretty close with a few minor alterations. Just remember that the main reason for dissatisfaction with hairstyling services is the insistence of a client to have her hair styled in a manner which goes against the natural inclination of her hair.

Okay. The consultation proceeds. You and the stylist are looking at your reflection in the mirror as he starts to brush your hair, this way, that way, to pull your hair to one side, brush it forward, brush it back. He has a bemused look on his face and he may be keeping up a line of chatter. He's getting not only an analytical feel for your hair and what it will do, but also this is where the artist comes in. He is getting an intuitive feeling and he is creating an aesthetic plan for how your hairstyle will be completed.

So, have a dialogue with whomever is going to style your hair. As hairstyling great Kenneth Battelle says: "If that person doesn't want to have a dialogue with you, get up out of the chair. I have clients who come in and sit down and say, 'Oh, you're so famous, do anything you want.' I don't want to do anything I want. You've got to be part of it. If you're not, you're never going to be happy." So the real pros agree. The word consultation means "to consult," "to deliberate," "to take counsel." This implies the relationship is equal. So now as the consultation proceeds, you and the stylist are going to continue to discuss the elements that will result in the final hairstyle.

It's all very well and good to say that you should be consulting with the hairstylist, but are you talking the same language? Star stylists John and Suzanne Chadwick point out that it's essential to learn basic hairstyling terms. As John Chadwick says, "If you go into a salon and ask for a blunt cut thinking you are asking for a bob, you're headed for trouble. A blunt cut simply means a haircutting technique. Even a layered cut can be a blunt cut. And, of course, a bob is a style where all hair is cut to the same length. So it's essential to learn basic terms. And most important—so that you will know what he/she is suggesting before it's too late."

These are terms used to describe different kinds of haircutting techniques:

- *Layering:* cutting the hair in different lengths to produce volume and create shape
- *Graduation:* a layered haircut
- *General graduation:* an all-over layering technique
- *Subtle graduation:* a limited use of layering or selective layering in one area
- *Blunt cut:* a haircut using scissors that helps to discourage split ends

Even when a style is cut in many layers the cutting technique may be a blunt cut. This is used to achieve a clean line and freely swinging hair. The opposite of a blunt cut is the razor cut—very popular years ago when highly teased hairstyles were in vogue, because the tapered ends obtained by this cutting technique allowed the hair to be shaped into teased hairstyles. Contemporary styling calls for blunt scissors cutting and that is probably what you will get with any contemporary haircut unless you and your stylist discuss the reasons for having a razor cut.

The Long and the Short of It

The heart of your styling consultation is this: how much change do you want as the final result of today's hairstyling? In other words, you and your stylist should be talking with two goals in mind: the results of today's styling—are you going for a *big* change, or are you aiming for a maintenance styling while you let your hair grow?

Transition Styling: If your Close-up analysis has shown you that you have been wearing your hair too short to be truly flattering, you want to embark on a transition styling that will keep your hair looking attractive while it grows long enough to be styled into your ultimate Close-up hairstyle. *So let your hairstylist know that you are not looking for the perfect hairstyle today, simply an interim style that will carry you through the next few months.* And your hairstylist can do so much to make your growing-out period an attractive one. These are a few of the styling tricks he/she can employ to turn that "it's driving me crazy and I'm going to get it all cut off anyway" growing-out style into something that is flattering and livable.

1 *Layering.* When layered hair is growing out, it quickly loses the original styling shape and becomes untidy and shaggy looking. The reason: hair does not all grow at the same rate. Some will grow faster and some slower, so the layers become uneven. The stylist may trim some of the under layers while letting the top ones grow out. Just be sure you both have a clear understanding that you are talking about a quarter of an inch trim to shape the layers and not a whole new layered style that takes you back to square one.

2 *Perms.* Think about having a body wave or curly perm. This will definitely give the look and feel of more hair while your hair's length is growing.

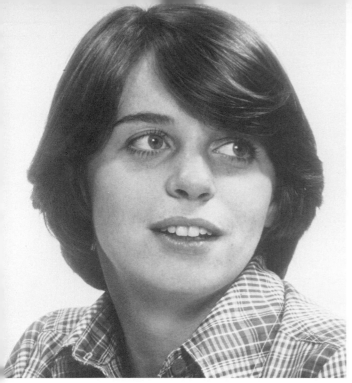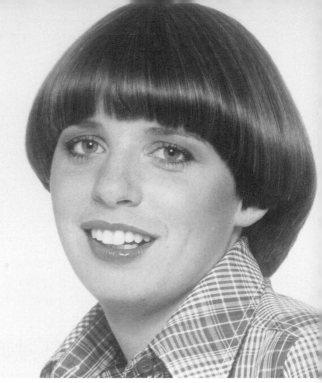

A transition styling keeps your Close-up image while your hair grows.

A transition style is essential when changing from a layered cut.

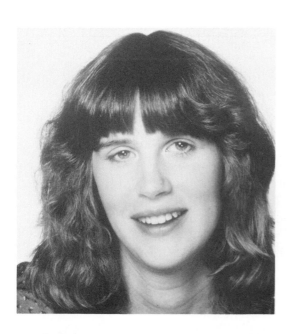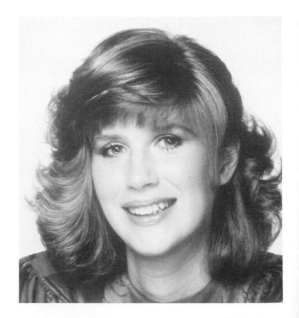

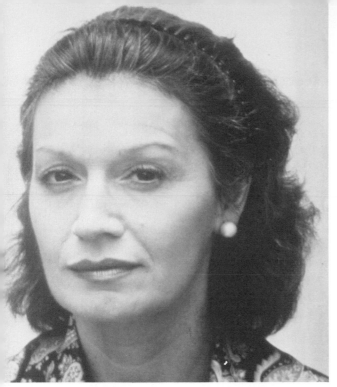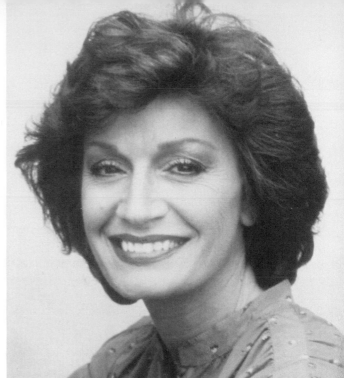

The ideal styling situation—hair that's long enough to create a beautiful new look.

3 *Bangs.* If you have been wearing bangs and you want them to grow out, have the stylist experiment with brushing them to the side, setting them on hot rollers or even twisting them into a little roll, secured with a hair ribbon or ornament.

But let's say that you have a good crop of hair for the stylist to work with. And so today you and the stylist are going to create that wonderful hairstyle that will complete your Close-up Portrait. This is where you have to get specific about length. As the stylist describes to you what he/she plans to do—and you have every right to expect that you will get a detailed description of what is going to happen to your precious hair—be sure to talk length in specific terms. Does he plan to cut one inch, one-half inch, one-quarter inch, and where will these lengths be on your head? How long will the hair be at the crown? How long will it be at the back of your neck? Don't feel shy about getting *specific*. A good hairstylist will be happy to talk in these terms. But what if you find that Mr. Z. brushes off your questions or that Miss L. says rather huffily, "Well really, short hair is *in* and all my clients love the cuts I do." In other words, if they're not willing to talk about your precious crop of hair, get right up out of that chair and go to the next stylist on your list. Remember, the theme of this hairstyling production is *your* ego, not theirs. And good stylists will want to please you. It's just a question of finding the middle ground between your personal and emotional needs and the professional advice that you are paying for.

Maintenance. The final element to be considered in your hairstyling consultation is the maintenance of the style that you will be getting. If you are really on a tight budget, choose a hairstyle that requires low maintenance, and share this information with your stylist.

The consultation is over. Let the styling begin.

All good professional haircuts will begin with freshly shampooed hair. Even if you have washed your hair the day before or even that morning, the stylist will want to work on your still-wet shampooed hair. There is another reason for this: in his/her evaluation of your hair, the stylist will be mentally noting what kinds of conditioners will enhance the quality of your hair and add to the final results of the styling. For example, does your coarse, wiry hair need a softening, silkening agent? Or would your fine, silky hair benefit from a volume-producing conditioner?

Okay. You're sitting in the stylist's chair listening to the mesmerizing clip-clip-clip of the styling scissors. What do you do now? You can become totally engrossed in the latest issue of *People* magazine, or you can keep up a steady line of chatter with the stylist about the movie you saw last weekend. Or, and this is the wisest course, you can pay attention to the progress of this hairstyle. If you don't like the way things are proceeding—if it looks as if your hair is going to be too long in the back or if your bangs appear to be embarking on a short short story—speak up. This is not to say that you should sit tensely in the styling chair watching every move with beady-eyed intensity. It simply means that you stay involved in the process and keep up a pleasant line of communication with your hairstylist. After all, the result that any good stylist is working for, the emotional payoff for these artists, is the thoroughly delighted client. Just remember that after the consultation comes concentration. *Concentrate* on what is happening as your hairstyle proceeds from shampoo to cut to the next step, which is . . .

The Finishing Touch

A beautiful hairstyle is composed of two parts: first, the expert cut—one that has a line and shape without the necessity of elaborate setting techniques—and second, the finishing touch. And drying your hair is the initial technique to guide your style into a flattering line and shape that will be part of the final picture. If you have always wielded your hair dryer with cavalier abandon, simply pointing the nozzle at your mop of wet hair and hoping for the best, now is the time to pay attention to the professional approach to hair drying.

The professional stylist will proceed to dry your hair in an orderly fashion, and you must do this too.

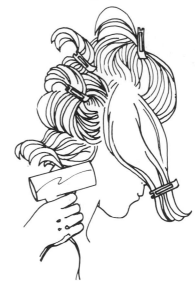

• Using a wide-toothed comb, he will gently comb out your hair. There will be few tangles because salons routinely use conditioners and rinses designed to detangle the hair and help avoid tugging and pulling the hair in its wet, weakened condition. This is a very important step in home hairstyling. Be sure to include appropriate conditioners and/or styling rinses in your daily shampoo schedule.

Professional drying techniques add the finishing touch to your hairstyle.

● Watch how the stylist divides your hair into four sections, the crown, the back, and the two sides, using long hair clips to keep these sections separated. When you dry your hair, copy his routine. Start by drying the back section, then the sides and finally the crown hair.

● Holding the brush in your left hand (if you are right-handed) place the brush underneath the hair close to the roots. Lift and guide, do not pull, the strand away from the head as, holding the dryer in your right hand, you direct the heat first to the roots, then to the middle of the strand and finally the end. Dry all hair in the same way. You'll finish by drying the crown hair. Notice how the professional stylist lifts and gently moves the crown hair in the opposite direction from the direction it grows? The lifting action creates the look of flattering volume and fullness.

Here are more professional drying tips:

● If hair is fine, long or color-lightened, towel it dry before working with your hand-held styling dryer.

● Speed up drying time of thick, coarse hair by using a hand-held dryer on wet hair.

● If your hair is naturally curly and you want to encourage the curl, blow-dry damp hair using the fingers to lift, shape and encourage the natural curls and waves. If you want to straighten naturally curly hair, blow it dry while it's very wet. This will discourage the waves and curls and give you more styling control.

Once the hair is dry, the stylist goes on to the final or finishing steps. There are several techniques that can be used. Each technique uses different beauty tools.

● *The round styling brush* used on ends to flip hair up or turn it under. Your stylist will probably use just one hand, and, with a casual flip of the wrist, turn the ends under while wielding the hair dryer to set the shape of the hair. You should probably use two hands. Put the hair dryer down and hold the round brush in one hand. With the other, wrap dried hair around the brush, then use a twisting motion to curl the hair up or under. Once the hair is in place, direct the hairdryer at the round brush. Turn the dryer off and hold the brush in place until the hair is completely curled. Use two hands to unwrap the hair from the round brush. Repeat this process wherever a flip-up or curl-under is desired. Use the round brush for bangs, too, using the same technique, if you want your bangs to curl under slightly. For short layered cuts, the round styling brush can be used to add lift and direction to longer crown hair and to bangs as described above.

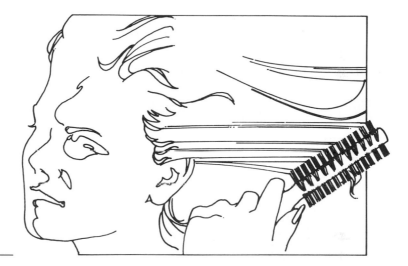

The round styling brush can be used to flip up hair ends or curl them under.

● *Curling irons* are the most creative of the electric curling appliances. They can be used to give a little extra lift to the crown hair, to sweep bangs to one side, to flip the ends of longer hair under or up, to twirl a curl into a tendril. If you want to make waves, this is an instant way to do it. Instant, yes, easy, no. I feel that curling irons take the most practice and dexterity. Still, they are well worth the time invested in practice. Watch your stylist carefully if he/she uses a curling iron to finish your hairstyle. Notice that he always *starts with dry hair.*

● *Electric rollers.* These instant hairsetters are the easiest way to create firm, long-lasting curls and luxuriant waves. Whatever your hair type there is an electric roller set designed to give you the most satisfying results. If your hair doesn't curl easily, the regular unit is for you. There are electric curler sets that have a water-mist feature which makes it easier to roll up your hair and creates a softer curl. The newest addition to the electric roller family is the velvet-covered heated roller that is especially kind to lightened or fine, silky hair.

After you have curled your hair with a curling iron or electric rollers, don't finish your hairstyling by gingerly combing your hair into place. Follow the knowledgeable technique of professional stylists.

After your curls have thoroughly cooled, your stylist will give your hair a final and thorough brushing. He may even ask you to bend over from the waist and brush down, starting at the back of your neck and working through all the hair. When you do this, let the brush roll through your hair—use a twist of the wrist—and lift hair up and out. Think of fluffing and blending your hairstyle so that it will flow into the styling line the finishing techniques have created.

Finally, your stylist will smooth your hair into shape with the brush. He may give you a tiny touch of back-combing (using a *brush*) to give a little lift at the crown. Watch how your stylist does this. You'll see that he just does one or two back-strokes near the hair's roots. No elaborate beehive techniques are allowed! If your hair is soft and fine, a quick spritz of hair spray will add the finishing touch and—voilà! Enjoy the mirror image that shows you the perfect frame for your Close-up Makeover.

Day 7 — Beauty Essence Workout: Your Declaration of Independence — Who Are You Trying to Please?

At this point in your Close-up Makeover, you'll see some big changes. In your looks, in your attitudes. And people will notice! Does this mean a bouquet of compliments for you? Absolutely! Still, some of the people in your life may need a little help in adjusting to the beautiful changes in you.

What about the reactions of your children? Younger children usually adore Close-up Makeover changes. "You were the prettiest Mommy at Parents' Night . . . and I was so proud." Teenagers can be something else. So often, any indication that Mother is a person, a real live woman, can be alarming and unsettling. The result—a negative and even hostile reaction from your teen. Face it. Your Close-up Makeover may not get the seal of approval from your teenager. After all, isn't that the essence of the teen years—a rejection of all that is adult?

But what about you? Your Close-up Makeover is bringing *you* rewards in terms of confidence, renewed self-awareness and a feeling of self-worth. (And let's be honest. Those payoffs may be long overdue. Right, Mother?) So, go for it! And let your teens learn a valuable lesson. Being an adult—and a mother—has some genuine visible rewards. Your teen may not be entirely comfortable with the beautiful changes in you, but he or she will *respect* you for being your best self. Not a bad tradeoff.

What about your friends? Most will be thrilled and fascinated by the subtle image changes your Close-up Makeover is creating. And they will probably want to know, in detail, what it is that you're doing to look so *marvelous*. In fact, your closest friends are probably sharing your Close-up Makeover program. (Remember, there is strength in numbers.)

But there may be other friends who are not quite so enthusiastic. They are the ones who want you to remain physically and emotionally "living in the old neighborhood." A successful and lasting makeover represents a statement of not only outer enhancement but also inner growth. Some friends and family are challenged and upset by any change at all. They feel uncomfortable.

The power of our own public's opinion cannot be underestimated. Maggie's story will show you what I mean. Maggie is an elegant, delightful woman who has recently divorced and now, after many months of emotional convalescence, is ready to go out, meet men and start a new romantic life. She has a large and loving circle of friends who see her as she has been to them for so many years—an elegant, conservative matron. While a new, younger, ageless image would rejuvenate Maggie's sexual confidence, her friends—ah, her friends—*they* can't take it. Each small attempt on Maggie's part to look and be different is greeted with disapproval by her loving friends. Maggie finds that maintaining the status quo wins strokes and approval from them. "Well, Maggie, I'm certainly glad that you're handling all these changes so sensibly." Or the flip side, "Good heavens, Maggie, isn't that dress a bit daring for the club dance?" So Maggie must choose: to shake up her life and quite possibly her friends and let her life move into new spheres—in other words, to "move into a new neighborhood"—or to get all her emotional sustenance in the old ways from her friends.

So, it may be necessary for you to "leave the old neighborhood" emotionally. You can go back for a visit, but you'll never live there again. In fact, if you've come this far in your Close-up Makeover, you've already moved out—and up! Your Close-up Makeover is an intensely personal form of self-expression. Who are you trying to please? The only right answer is *You.*

Eleven

DAY EIGHT

"It's a Wrap!"

That's TV talk for the successful completion of a TV spot. When all the many elements—on-camera talent, props, lighting, sound—come together to produce a memorable visual image, a segment clicks, and "It's a wrap." Today, on Day 8, you're going to wrap it up. You're going to put together all of the elements that will complete your makeover. So far we've been working on close-ups, perfecting your image from the neck up. But now we're going to concentrate on long shots and the clothes that complete the image you project from head to toe.

Clothes definitely play a supporting role in a successful Close-Up Makeover. There are two reasons for this.

First, facial impact is the number-one dynamic in your image. If hair, makeup and facial expressions are all positive and attractive, the simplest of clothes will be effective. To quote Edith Head, "I always design for close-ups because that's where all of the meaningful and exciting action in any plot takes place."

And second, most of us interact with people in situations where we're being seen from the waist up, in close-ups. Think about it. Aren't we usually seen at a desk, at a table, or standing close enough to people—

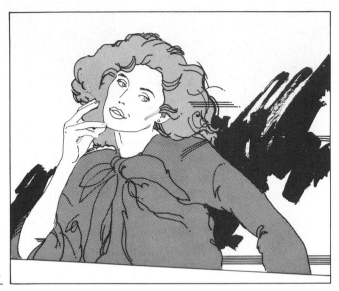

*Our personal audience
usually sees us in Close-ups.*

that is, two or three feet away—so that they are concentrating on us from
the neck up rather than seeing the total image or the long shot?

It's not that clothes are totally unimportant; on the contrary, the
right clothes can effectively point up your best features and also dramatize your total image. But, they must play a secondary role. Yet most
women place too much emphasis on the clothes they wear and too little
on their hair and makeup. They're paying too much for clothes—in
terms of attention and money.

How to Put Star Quality into Real-Life Clothes

Here are some simple rules to follow in creating your wardrobe to fit
your Close-up Makeover personality.

1. Never wear anything that you don't love.   More isn't necessarily better. Having lots of blah clothes that don't do anything for you, either visually or emotionally, will make you feel like an "extra" every time. Now, on Day 8, is the time to ruthlessly discard anything that doesn't make you look and *feel* terrific. Your goal? To have everything in your closet — from bathing suits to blazers—be a super-flattering, ego-boosting Look. A cluttered closet so often represents a cluttered, confused self-image. Today's Beauty Essence Workout shows how to clean out your closet so all your clothes are star-quality.

2. Never wear anything that isn't flattering to you.   What we love isn't necessarily flattering. Somewhere along the line, one must make a choice, and flattery, in my book, must come first. Of course, the looks you love and the looks that flatter will not always conflict. Quite the opposite. Feedback from friends, acquaintances and even strangers gives us a continuing evaluation of what's fabulously flattering. But to remind yourself of the styles, silhouettes and lines that are most becoming to you, rummage through that mini-boutique that resides in your closet and pick out the blouses, jackets, skirts and dresses that always get rave reviews. Analyze these clothing items to discover the design elements that make them so flattering. In this situation, your best friend is your full-length mirror. Try on your wardrobe and, using the same Objectivision analysis that has worked so successfully for your face, see what your favorite clothes do for your figure. Does that long, lean tunic worn over a straight skirt camouflage very effectively your slightly chunky waist? Perhaps your favorite red skirt with the slight gathers at the top creating a dirndl effect is one of the most talked-about items in your wardrobe, not only because of the color but also because the style effectively camouflages that hip bulge you hate.

Obviously, sticking doggedly to the tried and true looks you've worn for years isn't the point. It's essential, in completing your makeover, that you be open to the *new.* A try-on shopping spree can help you loosen up and find out what's new and still right for you.

Here's the idea. Every season, make a date with yourself to take a

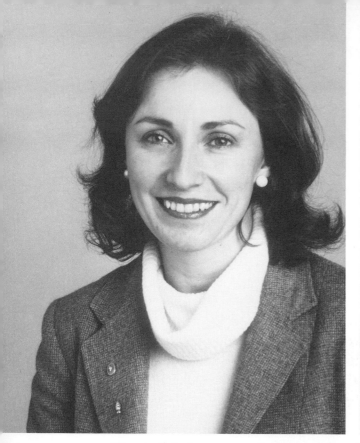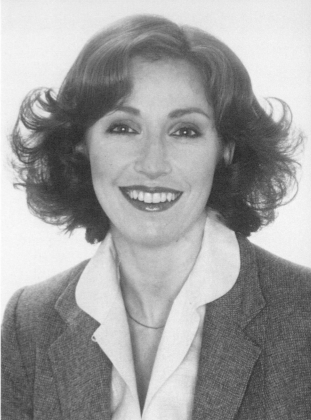

The spotlight is on you—that's why clothes play a supporting role in your Close-up.

shopping trip during which you will try on *only* those styles and colors that are part of the newest fashion themes. While flattery always gets the nod over fashion, the two don't necessarily conflict. *Get over this idea.* The biggest image mistake I see women making is to become victims of "lazy eye." They become locked into a look that worked for them once, and their visual perception has stuck in neutral for five, ten or even twenty years. The lazy-eye philosophy is built on this (erroneous) assumption: "Fashion changes. What's becoming to me doesn't." Wrong!

Every fashion season there will be at least one completely contemporary, fashionable look that will be flattering to you. And the long-term fashion themes—those changes that cover about a five- to seven-year span—will always have some basic silhouette, some fashionable design elements that will look terrific on you.

But there's something else involved here. Because fashion is composed of a series of subtle changes in proportion and accent, you must learn not just to look, but to *see.* You must continually stimulate and educate your eyes to new lines, colors, proportions and, ultimately, to a new visual message.

3. The educated eye. Fashion magazines are excellent sources of realistic fashion information. Yes, I know—a cursory glance at the improbable photos of flakey fashions photographed on thirteen-year-old models makes you wonder if these mags have any relationship to the real world at all. But, armed with a bit of knowledge, you can use the fashion mags as an instructive guide to putting yourself into livable, wearable, fashionable and flattering clothes. The editorial pages of *Vogue, Harper's, Mademoiselle* and *Glamour* spell out very clearly what's new and wearable if you know the trick of translating their flowery language into real-life terms. Here are examples:

- *Silhouettes.* "Skirts are gentler, softer, longer . . . pants are fuller on top . . . tapering at the ankle." (*Vogue*, October 1983)
- *Hemlines.* "One thing that's new—a longer, narrower silhouette often (but not always) in new longer lengths." (*Vogue*, December 1983)
- *Colors.* ". . . gray, the color of the future. Smartly modern and wonderfully practical. . . . Gray and white—the coolest combination." (*Harper's Bazaar*, March 1982)
- *Accessories.* "The key word in accessories now is soft, sculptural brass cuffs . . . washed with sultry violet or mauve tones . . . waist and hip wraps in the softest leathers and suedes, even in woven scarves . . ." (*Harper's Bazaar*, March 1982)

Look for statements like those above to provide clues about the very latest trends. Other guides to "what's new" are found in the windows and display islands of your favorite store. The mannequins will display the newest complete looks. Check out the design elements listed above, paying special attention to colors and accessories. Really study all the details that create the look—like the placement of a pin; the play of color and texture in two scarves that have been twisted to form a new-looking belt; the charm of a blouse and skirt and jacket in color-melting layers.

Armed with these guides, you can go to the next step in creating star-quality clothes.

4. *Dress for total impact.*   We've all seen her: the woman whose concept of herself is so complete, so integrated, that every aspect of her image is part of a harmonious and expressive theme. It may be type-casting, but it's an effect that is as riveting as a spotlight. This total impact is the essence of star quality, and *simplicity* is the key.

All star-quality clothes have great simplicity, and interestingly, simplicity translates to authority. The simplest costumes express presence and self-confidence because they enhance rather than overpower your image. The outfit that is too gimmicked up with accessories, too confused with colors and prints, detracts from you as an individual and may telegraph the message that you are not secure and confident.

The clothes that I choose to complete my television makeovers usually consist of a simple blouse and classic skirt or a dress—always very simple but in a flattering color. And then we add accessory accents. I recommend this approach to completing your makeover because it is not a big strain on your budget, and after all, you are still getting used to your new image. Just as I advised you to do for everything from the neck up, use small subtle steps to develop your new wardrobe.

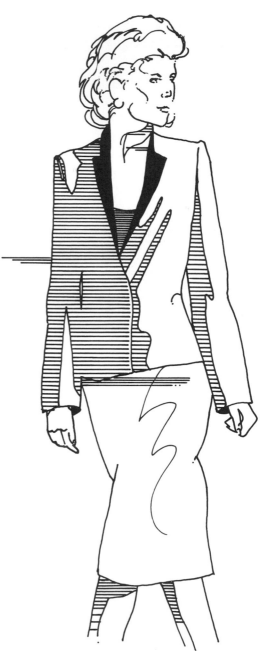

Clothes with star quality make you feel terrific.

However, in putting together the one perfect outfit that will complete your Close-up Makeover and that you will wear in your "after" picture, it's important to think in terms of completing the Close-up Portrait that you have chosen. You get star-quality looks by following your Close-up theme in every element of your total image. The components of hair, makeup, clothes and accessories should express the overall theme you have chosen. This does not mean a relentless pursuit of mixey-matchey perfection—the green suede purse that exactly matches the green suede shoe. That's a fashion approach that is boring and predictable and belongs in the chorus line.

No, we'll work with the simplest elements, the way that costume designers do it—color and a few accessories—to create one perfect outfit that expresses *you*.

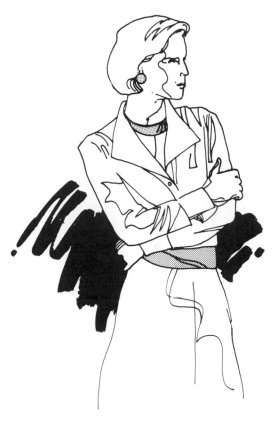

Use separates creatively and turn them into accessories.

You: In Living Color

I'd like to suggest a color philosophy that is a popular approach to costume design on stage and screen. Instead of having a closet whose theme song appears to be "Somewhere Over the Rainbow," why not choose one or two color themes. Pare down the number of colors in your wardrobe to two or three basics that will all combine. Then use two or three accent colors in the form of blouses, jackets, and accessories. The result? A wardrobe that has drama and authority. What's more, it's a low-budget plan with big-budget impact.

Karen Cadle, chic producer of "Hour Magazine," follows her own version of color paring that is effective and time-saving. "I stick to three or four color themes and whenever I shop I simply buy shades in one of four themes—beige, camel, wine and peach are my current favorites. It makes dressing so simple because you simply reach in the closet and everything goes with everything else."

Geraldine Stutz, president of Henri Bendel specialty store in New York, explains her fashion philosophy vis-à-vis color: "My wardrobe is based on black and white with a few color accents. And I wear white whatever the season. My favorite designer's white is not white-white, but an ivory. You need a large chunk of it for black." A typical daytime look for Stutz would be white and black worn with shots of strong bright color—a coral turban and coral and ivory necklace and cuffs.

Another tip from the costume world of the theater is to go easy on prints, plaids and stripes. Use them as you would spice—an addition but not the whole meal. The reason for this is that patterns and prints tend to be very interesting in themselves and detract from the individual. Not surprisingly, people become visually engrossed in prints that feature, say, a multicolored crested cockatoo rampant on a forest of banana leaves, and they don't notice you at all!

Here's a short-cut to finding the colors that turn the spotlight on you. I call it the "blouse method." Look in your closet and find a skirt and a jacket or a pair of pants and a jacket that are basic in color. And then shop for a very wonderful blouse that will go with them. Choose a blouse in your favorite color or choose something that you've never worn before. Look through those racks and racks of colorful blouses and try on at least five different colors. As you work your way through the racks, be aware of the variety of shades in each color family. While that poppy red silk T-shirt may not be right for you, the rose-red blouse next to it may be as flattering as a diamond necklace. Try it—you'll like it. Now is the time to go for something that's fun and new and different. Often women find that bringing color into their lives through the hair and makeup changes in the first seven days of their Close-up Makeover allows them to see an entirely new color palette emerging.

Another color approach that will add star quality to the simplest, most budget-conscious outfit is to immerse yourself in one fabulously flattering shade. Think lilac. Turquoise blue. Shocking pink. Even black and white can create color impact. This is a never-miss approach that I often use to create one perfect outfit for the women in my TV makeovers. Nowhere do we get more beauty value for our dollar than through the medium of flattering color.

Here is how I put together the one perfect outfit for Vickie. She was about forty and when photographed for her "before" picture, had mousey salt-and-pepper hair and a pale complexion which appeared even more sallow because of the beige pant suit she was wearing. The day after Vickie's salon makeover, her hair had been transformed to a soft, flattering apricot blonde. Pale skin had suddenly become peachy and creamy in tone. And the makeup accents I had directed further increased the effect of a golden peachy aura. A silk blouse in a melting peach color and a deeper peach linen skirt were the basis for her "after" picture's one perfect outfit. The melting, delicious colors of her skirt and blouse blended with her Close-up color scheme to make a dramatic million-dollar look. A faux-ivory necklace, classic button earrings and ivory-colored pumps (the result of a shopping trip through Vickie's own closet) combined with pale bone stockings completed the outfit. How simple and basic can you get? But remember: a six-carat diamond solitaire is simple and basic, too.

Accessories for Close-ups and Long Shots

A simple blouse and skirt can, at first glance, be a rather bland dish. That's why it's essential to add the spice of carefully chosen accessories. Here is my recipe. The old-fashioned, timid idea of accessorizing an outfit—taking a simple blouse and skirt and adding a single gold chain—doesn't make it at all. In the contemporary fashion scene, accessories *are* the look-makers of fashion. When the foundation of real clothes consists of separates, simple tops and bottoms that work interchangeably, it's the accessories that create the drama. They have to be *now* and they have to be *right*. Every time you move things around—wear a shirt as a jacket to make a suit; layer two silky skirts for a tone-on-tone color effect; top a straight skirt and T-blouse with a coat dress, unbuttoned and worn as an updated duster—you are creating a look.

Notice that when you're dressing in pieces, almost anything can be an accessory. So think beyond the usual scarves, bracelets and belts. To really understand the current approach to accessorizing, broaden your thinking to include jackets and important blouses. Even purses and shoes can be considered accessories when they are in bright or unexpected colors or fabrics. Remember, an accessory doesn't have to combine with *everything* in your closet. If it transforms two or three outfits into something special, it's earned its place.

Scarves, necklaces and earrings will focus attention on your Close-ups. Size is important when it comes to choosing jewelry. If you have a large facial area, wide cheekbones or prominent features, be sure to choose chunky important earrings—tiny little earbobs will make your face unflatteringly heavy by comparison. Luckily, big dramatic earrings are big news in the '80s. What if you have a delicate facial structure? You can still be in fashion; just choose a smaller version of these dramatic earring styles, one that will look important in relation to your personal proportions.

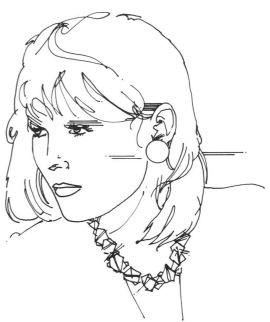

Keep jewelry in proportion.

Exotic chunky necklaces are the perfect accent for simple blouses and skirts. Semi-precious stones, unusual hand-carved beads, twisted and plaited cords and heavy strands of shells are all exciting looks that are in fashion. But suppose you have a long, long neck, or a short and chunky one. Then size isn't as important as placement. A long string of beads will make a long neck look swanlike all right—but who wants to look like a swan? If your neck is short and wide, don't wear that chunky choker either. It will just make your neck look shorter and wider. A dramatic bulky necklace that falls several inches below your collar bone and covers the sides of your neck will make a wide neck look better in every way. The chunky necklace will make your sturdy neck appear delicate by comparison.

Many women have a combination problem—a long slender neck that is wide at the base. This is easy to camouflage. Never wear an unadorned neckline is the first rule. Use a bulky necklace or a loosely knotted scarf to cover the wide base of your neck and accent its delicate length.

More neckline tips: in a fashion era of wide shoulders, big flyaway sleeves and wide, soaring collars, check out the effect of all this width on your neck proportion. Does your slender neck look like a periscope rising timidly out of this froth of sleeve and collar? If so, you could add bulk (a counterbalancing proportion) by wearing a very impor-

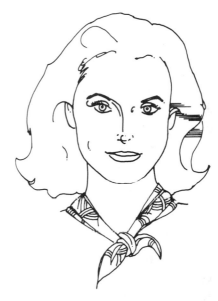

Use a necklace or scarf to camouflage a slender neck that is broad at the base.

tant bulky choker at the neckline. Or you may decide to forget the whole thing and wear a T-shirt instead. So much for Close-ups, now let's take a look at those long shots.

Slenderness may be your problem below the hemline. So many women who wish they were small in the hip and thigh area have surprisingly delicate calves. They look like matchsticks when paired with bulky, chunky or brightly colored shoes. Slender legs that are very tan or that sport tan-colored stockings worn with light-colored shoes will make any woman look like Minnie Mouse for sure. Instead, choose the most delicate narrowly styled shoes you can find. Light-colored stockings, textured stockings, or opaque rather than sheer dark stockings will make your legs look more rounded.

If heavy legs are your problem, they will always look longer and more slender if they are color-keyed to the hem of your skirt. For example, a navy blue skirt with sheer rather than opaque navy blue stockings, navy blue shoes. The elongating effect of this one-color sweep from waist to shoe works with both light and dark colors and is a favorite technique used by costume designers in film and television to create an effect of height and slenderness. In fact, the slenderizing effect of matching shoe and stocking tones is so universally flattering that I can recommend beige or bone shoes teamed with matching stockings as an all-year-round, always-flattering basic for every woman.

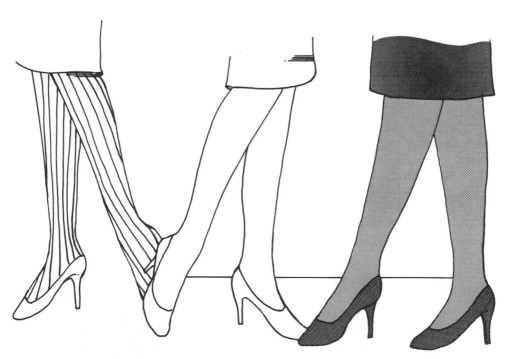

Thin legs appear rounded in bright-colored or textured stockings. Heavy legs look long and slender when color-keyed to skirt hem.

This Is Your Life: Dress for It

With clothes and accessories completing the picture, you have painted in the background and chosen the frame to make your Close-up Portrait complete. Because each Portrait represents a distinct beauty temperament and the resultant life style, I will not describe the one perfect outfit for your Close-up Portrait in terms of specific clothing items. That's for you to choose. The Alluring Beauty may wish to create one perfect outfit that she would wear to a cocktail party or for an intimate dinner for two. The Casual Beauty may be interested in putting together an outfit she will wear to her jogging club.

And is it important to have one perfect look to wear jogging, for example? Absolutely. Remember the philosophy behind a star-quality wardrobe is this: never wear anything that you don't love.

Here are brief scenarios to guide you in plotting your One Perfect Outfit.

THE TRULY NATURAL BEAUTY

Natural colors will predominate in any Truly Natural Wardrobe. I mean not only colors that relate to nature—all shades of brown, beige, rust, green, mulberry, flower colors of course—but also colors that are the result of natural dyes rather than the sophisticated chemical dye shades. Cotton and linen fabrics in their natural tone-on-tone shades of bone and cream, or alpaca sweaters in shades ranging from gray to camel to brown are good examples. Similarly, fabrics will be textured in feeling and hand-crafted, possibly with a charmingly irregular finish that bespeaks the hand rather than the machine.

Ethnic themes are so appropriate for Truly Natural Beauties because they represent a way of life far distant from our industrial civilization, a way of life that is closer to nature, closer to the earth. So any native products—cottons from Haiti, crinkled silks from India, hand-loomed wools from the sheer mountains of Bolivia—all of these moods will be expressive of the Truly Natural Beauty. Accessories would include jewelry in wood or faux-ivory. A wonderful source of remarkable and unique ethnic jewelry, all at very reasonable prices, is any large museum. If you don't have access to museums, their catalogs are a marvelous source of unusual jewelry that will complete your Truly Natural Portrait.

Pitfalls in creating the total image for Truly Natural Beauties are these: when combined with the subtleties of natural fabrics and colors, your aversion to any artifice in makeup and hair coloring can make the Truly Natural Beauty very colorless indeed. Consider hair coloring in the form of very natural sunstreaks and perhaps add face coloring—blushers, a bit of eye makeup, a touch of lip color. And remember, if you include strong color in your one perfect outfit but keep your extremely subtle, underplayed coloring in your makeup and hair, your clothing will totally overshadow the most important element in this picture—your face. And that's not natural!

THE CASUAL BEAUTY

The essence of your one perfect outfit, and ultimately your Casual Beauty wardrobe, is the classic or preppy look. This means a complete design philosophy in clothing comprised of natural fabrics—silk, linen, wool, cotton—in firm, crisp, shape-retaining fabrics. Very little softness is seen in terms of color, texture or fabric weight.

Many of the same colors and textures that are seen in the Natural Beauty's wardrobe will find a place in the closet of the Casual Beauty, but with this difference. All clothing elements have a feeling of control and discipline—the same attitudes that give the Casual Beauty her athletic prowess and list of accomplishments. However, in terms of color, there are other standard colors that will find a place in her one perfect outfit and ultimately in her wardrobe. These would include red-white-and-blue combinations, bright pink, tulip yellow, parrot or Bermuda green.

For an overview of Casual Beauty dressing, I suggest Talbott's catalog (1-800-225-8200). Use this catalog for actually ordering the items for your one perfect outfit, or for getting an idea of the Casual Beauty's image. You'll quickly see that shapes are tailored, simple and classic in clothing; shoes are pumps, little Papagallo flats, spectators, penny loafers, and classic Spalding tennies for casual wear. Jewelry is (or looks like) the real thing: gold chains, pearls, Cartier tank watches, antique jewelry of all kinds.

But Casual Beauties must be careful of a too-tailored, no-nonsense image. Wash-and-wear haircuts, minimal makeup and tailored classic clothes add up to a boring, if not downright formidable, image. So avoid that boring, slightly unfeminine "play-to-win" girl's look by choosing classics with a flair. Ralph Lauren's argyle cardigan, for example, in non-classic turquoise, peach and lilac worn with a simple silk shirt and softly tailored skirt in creamy white will give a Casual Beauty "Great Gatsby" glamour.

THE CONTEMPORARY BEAUTY

The one perfect outfit for our Contemporary Beauty probably reflects the most outstanding aspect of her life style—the fact that she is a successful working woman. Still, I'm in strong disagreement with John Malloy's *Dress for Success* mini-man approach to the working uniform of the contemporary woman.

Although tailored, unfussy clothes are appropriate and effective for most business situations, the defeminizing, oppressive effect of men's-wear gray, tailored three-piece suits, sensible pumps and an attaché case simply doesn't work in the '80s. Certain colors can be called power colors—those familiar grayed, dull colors that seem to deny not only sensuality but even humanity. But the Contemporary Beauty should express not only her professionalism but also her essential female self by using power basics—black, navy, gray—and the power intellectuals—grayed-greens, burgundies, brown—with bright, emotional colors. Is a touch of daffodil yellow or a dash of hyacinth pink an effective component of power dressing? Yes. The solution is to combine the bright, emotional, humanistic colors with power basics. But the essential point is that the power colors should always predominate. For example, take this combination:

White wool jacket and skirt
Yellow/pink/white flowered blouse
Opaque white stockings
Yellow kid pumps

Certainly a delightful spring look, but too soft and gentle. Definitely not a professional look. Rather, combine brights with power colors in this way:

White wool jacket
Black skirt
Daffodil yellow silk shirt
Opaque white stockings (or sheer black)
Black kid pumps

Strong contrast with vital brights keeps the power going, but with a springtime, feminine difference. Still, the power colors must always be present.

The Contemporary Beauty's one perfect outfit would be chosen from finely textured fabrics—silky gabardine, broadcloth, possibly a very fine flannel. The subliminal message is that these fabrics are the result of generations of technical excellence; these colors are the product of complex dyeing techniques. And all design elements are subtle, sophisticated, civilized. In other words, this is the polar opposite of the theme of the Truly Natural Beauty, which includes charmingly irregular handcrafted finishes.

THE DESIGNING BEAUTY

Your one perfect outfit as well as your wardrobe will express fashion at its best. The challenge for you as a Designing Beauty is to be aware of the fashion options that are open to you now that your Close-up Makeover has given you confidence and the awareness that you can indeed express the fashion that you love and that you find so fascinating. If you feel a bit unsure about your ability to wear the latest fashions, remember the comment of Mainbocher, one of America's greatest designers: "A woman can wear anything with authority if she understands it." Designing Beauties always know the difference between fad and fashion. Fashionable clothes are always wearable. They needn't be classic, but they're never shocking as fads often are. True fashion changes gradually and fashion trends are always concerned with proportion. Fad is fashion taken to the max. Fads are a fun and inexpensive way of adding a right-now look to more perennial and classic fashions. The most accepted way to use them is to avoid gimmicky costume looks and choose instead fad colors and accessories in the form of belts, jewelry and scarves to add impact to classic backgrounds. Here are some recipes for spicing up your wardrobe from fashion's leaders. "I love accessories," says Oscar de la Renta in *"W,"* "but they have to be either minimal or extravagant, never middle of the road." Bill Blass echoes this philosophy: "With bold clothes, jewelry has to have authority. Even with pearls, you need six ropes right down to the knee. Otherwise they get lost." You get the idea. No timid, little dabs of accessory magic. If you're going to do it, *do* it.

The Designing Beauty's one perfect outfit will express the newest daring skirt lengths or the newest fashionable silhouette. She will express this silhouette in current fad colors and use amusing, innovative, off-beat accessories to give her design image *her* label.

Designing Beauties should beware of too much accent on fashion and too little attention to *you.* Some women, in effect, are wearing so many labels they've forgotten their own name. Joan Rivers is a perfect example of the power of fashion to create glamour. But her strong personality is in little danger of being overpowered by any dress. Just be sure, Designing Beauties, that you have a knowledgeable dialogue with your fashionable wardrobe so that *you* retain all the best lines.

THE ALLURING BEAUTY

The clothes of the Alluring Beauty, like her makeup and hairstyle, express one strong message: I am Woman. This doesn't mean that the Alluring Beauty arrives for every social situation dressed like a Playboy Bunny. Not at all. The truly successful Alluring Beauty knows that woman's greatest asset is man's imagination, and she uses subtle symbols to get the message across. And because love relationships almost always involve a combination of opposite emotions—passion and tenderness, flirtation and aloofness, aggression and passivity—so the visual symbols that the Alluring Beauty chooses often appear in opposites. Let's look at some of these elements.

Robert Herrick said, "A sweet disorder in the dress kindles in clothes a wantonness." Soft, flowing, slippy-slidey garments or clothes that are partially unfastened to reveal a bit of flesh are always sexy. Tennis shoes, jeans and a sweatshirt may not sound like a very alluring outfit, but if the jeans are tight-fitting to reveal the figure, and the sweatshirt has an oversized neckline that permits it to slip and slide invitingly over one shoulder, the image is definitely one of seduction. An elegant Grecian-styled evening dress knotted on one shoulder will still create erotic fantasies in the nearest male. If he unties the shoulder knot, voilà! Instant You!

Interestingly, very covered-up clothes also have plenty of allure. High-necked, long-sleeved garments give an enticing hint of the woman inside, if the fabric is soft, draping, and figure-revealing. Tight, buttoned-up, laced-up clothes are a real turn-on, as any Victorian gentleman would pantingly tell you.

The most sensual aspect of any garment is the material of which it is made. That's why the most alluring fabrics you can wear are silky, satiny, soft, and smooth, or warm, velvety, furry finishes, implying an animal nature beneath. In fact, wearing animal skins in the form of suede, leather or fur will tell the world you are a "foxy" lady indeed.

What else is sexy? Colors, of course, send a powerful emotional message. Red is the color of passion, and in the psychology of the color lexicon, black too has always been highly touted as a passionate hue. But I agree with Bob Mackie, TV's premier designer who has created sensational costumes for everyone from Barbra Streisand to Liza Minnelli to Cher: "White is the color of glamour and sex." Unless your personal color scheme is very pale, I nominate white, ivory, cream—the moon shades, as I call them—as being super-sexy colors. Of course, any color that is extremely flattering to you will add to your allure.

A final word about alluring colors, and this takes us back to the attraction of opposites that is often a basic plot element in any red-hot romance: when you are buying an extremely seductive item—a clinging silk jersey dress, a satin, off-the-shoulder blouse, a pair of leather jeans—choose these obviously sexy clothes in a nonsexy color. For example, choose that silk jersey dress in gray, brown, green, deep blue or beige rather than red.

Amusing and playful accessories are also alluring. One of my personal favorites is a pair of bold gold earrings in the form of lightning bolts. I wear them as one dramatic accent with an otherwise tailored or businesslike outfit. Worn to a reception or cocktail party, these earrings are always a springboard for light conversation and a fun and not-so-subtle statement of an electric temperament.

The sexiest item of clothing that any woman wears is, hands down, shoes. Delicate foot-flattering pumps, high heels, strappy sandals that reveal the foot, and, of course, playful shoes in bright colors, fun fabrics, or those sporting feminine bows or flowers—all of these styles will create an alluring impact in your wardrobe and in your one perfect outfit.

Seductive, alluring clothing and accessories must look expensive and luxurious. A cheap, red satin off-the-shoulder blouse is impossibly tarty and sleazoid. It's not a whisper, but a shout. However, a very expensive, subtly styled red satin blouse could be wonderful.

One of the most effective accessories that any woman can wear is her perfume. No one understands this more completely than the Alluring Beauty and here, *expensive* is the key word. Always wear the very best in fragrance. And subtlety works in the area of perfume as it does in color choice. According to Dr. Ivan Popov, rejuvenation expert of the Jet Set and an authority on aroma therapy, certain perfumes can indeed drive your man to turn off the Johnny Carson Show and turn his attention to you. According to Dr. Popov, the scents that can definitely stimulate his erogenous zones are jasmine and roses, but the doctor warns that they must be the natural substances in order to be sexually stimulating. "Joy" takes top honors in the department, but "Halston," "Adolfo," and "Bal à Versailles" are also candidates for scentsational come-ons.

Image overkill for the Alluring Beauty comes in too much of a good thing. If the style is sexy, the fabric sexy, the colors overpowering, the perfume engulfing, the message is "Hello, sailor!" Sexy but *subtle* is the right idea.

THE AGELESS BEAUTY

The Ageless Beauty will maintain her timeless look by studying the Close-up Portrait guides for the Designing Beauty and the Alluring Beauty, taking elements from both of these and applying them to her own wardrobe. The biggest challenge for her is to watch out for stereotyping.

The Ageless Beauty *must* avoid the too-timid look. Add a bit of drama through accessories and flattering colors. Conservative, safe clothes in neutral colors will make you look like your own grandmother— safe, safe, safe. From coast to coast, that's the boring theme of fashion for so many mature women. Instead of those Mama bags—huge purses with double handles—and conservative pumps with sensible heels, choose shoes, bags and accessories with some punch and excitement. And remember, colors should enliven rather than embalm!

Accent your femininity in every subtle ladylike way. Let your clothes stress that you are Woman. In choosing your one perfect outfit and ultimately your Close-up wardrobe, remember that fashion is the mature woman's best friend. Fashionable clothes tell the world you're not living in the past. And looking current keeps you looking young and feeling ageless, as well as having a stimulating effect, forcing you to look at yourself and the world around you with new awareness.

Day 8 — Beauty Essence Workout

Off with the old! By now, on Day 8, the time and effort you have put into your Close-up Makeover is paying big dividends. Visually you're getting plenty of positive feedback from family, friends and co-workers, and from your own Magic Mirror. Yes, something is definitely happening. You are developing a stronger sense of your image, a sense of who you are, than you have had for a long time. I urge you today to do a bit of self-analysis. Think of how the changes in your image, something that is immediately visible to you, are helping you to become aware of inner changes. The desire to express your best self is always an outer manifestation of inner growth and development. *Be proud of yourself.* The actions that you have taken to create your new image should signal to you that many of your dreams are absolutely possible. The challenge for you now is to catch hold of this new reality. That's why it's important today to get rid of excess baggage that ties you to former limiting attitudes about yourself. Which brings us to a very mundane spot—the door to your very own closet.

Today I want you to be ruthless and pare down the contents of that closet so that only the clothes that are expressive of *you* remain. When we really get to it, you will recognize that fully half of the clothes in your closet are never worn at all. They're just clanking chains reminding you of shopping mistakes or outgrown images. If you're really serious about expressing the real you, I challenge you to clean out and organize your closet. Trust me. You'll feel better and you'll look better once you know that everything hanging on your racks is wearable, updated, but most important, expressing your beauty essence.

Let's get started. The materials you'll need are paper, pen, and several large cardboard cartons.

1 Start with one section of your closet at a time—the job simply becomes more manageable this way and you won't find yourself overwhelmed and discouraged. In fact, if you are a real pack rat, promise yourself that you will work with just one or two feet of the clothing rack per clean-out session.

2 Designate each of three cartons for clothes you will throw or give away, clothes that need attention in order to become wearable, and clothes that need a "partner." The clothes in your closet that are completely wearable you will lay out on the bed.

3 This is the real cold-turkey treatment, so we're going to deal immediately with clothes that are to be thrown away. I know it's a trauma to give away items that you once paid a lot for or that were once your favorites, but look really closely at each item as you remove it from your closet. Is it a bit tatty, a bit shop-worn, does it look out of date and out of sync with your present life? What is that old picture frame going to do to the beautiful new portrait you have just painted? Get rid of it and put it in the carton marked GIVE AWAY.

4 As you analyze each item, see if it can be used out of its usual context. In a recent "Hour Magazine" makeover, we used the red wool scarf from a model's outdated raincoat as a stunning belt on her basic gray wool dress. If you're agonizing over keeping something or getting rid of it, ask: did I use this item in the last year? If you haven't worn those blue-checked pants in the last year, why not? Try them on and take a look: (1) they don't fit; (2) they really are too old and worn-looking; or (3) they need some attention. Could they be shortened to look more fashionable? In that case put them into box #2 marked NEEDS ATTENTION. Be ruthless here. Would those pants need the full-time services of a Parisian couturier to whip them into wearable shape? Then forget it and get rid of them.

5 When you try on that pair of blue-checked pants, you may find that they fit beautifully and are not too worn, but they've been hanging in your closet because they need another item to complete the look. In that case, toss them into the third box which is marked NEEDS A PARTNER.

6 Work through your closet in this manner. Pay special attention to the clothes that are stacking up on the bed. Do you really love each look there and does it represent one or more of the Close-up Portraits that express the real you? Do the active parts of your wardrobe really express all facets of your personality, the realities of your life? It's terribly important to know you look your best anytime, anywhere—in the boardroom, on the tennis court, reading the Sunday paper in jeans and a color-flattering sweatshirt. Everything you wear becomes a personal statement about who you are. You're not only telling your audience who you are, but most important, *you are expressing your beauty essence to yourself.*

Analyzing the wearable clothes in your closet may also show you an out-of-balance attitude in your life. For example, a woman who discovers that she has two or three very special outfits to wear when she goes out but that her daily wardrobe is composed of worn, outmoded, boring basics, has found out something very important about her life. She has allowed her daily life to become boring and unfulfilling and has settled for a few rare high points interspersed between the gray valleys. Could this woman be you? Then I say to you: listen, every day of your life is important. No, make that priceless. Start now to build a wardrobe that expresses the best of you every single day.

Twelve

DAY NINE

It's Your Move: Body Language and Beautiful Hands

By Day 9 in your Close-up Makeover, you're going to find that you are moving toward a more confident body language, that unspoken, persuasive dialogue that tells the world so much about you.

This confident new element in *your* image is developing surely, naturally, without any conscious effort on your part. These are some of the positive and very attractive changes you can expect to see in your overall image impact:

1 Improved posture. It's no coincidence that posture is another word for attitude or state of mind. As you progress through the steps of your Close-up Makeover, your attitude about yourself is changing, dramatically. And you'll find that, just naturally, you'll stand taller, head held high, shoulders back, with lifted chest. As my favorite drama coach was fond of reminding us, "Remember, the 'lead with your chest' stance is the mark of beauty queens and winners in all fields—both male and female. The sunken, lowered chest posture is the stance of the defeated, the weak, the losers of this world." Your makeover will make you feel like a queen, and you'll move like one.

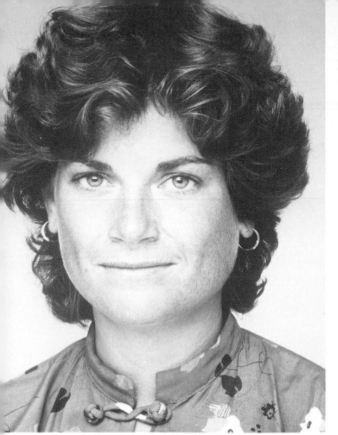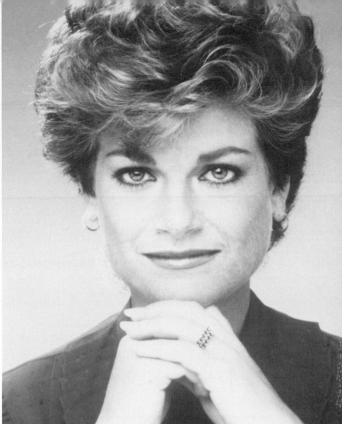

Right along with your facial expression, your hands continually reveal your emotions.

2 Your walk will become carefree and dynamic—more of a confident stride. Good. Go with it. Swing your legs freely and smoothly from the hip joint, and step right out—into that great future that awaits you.

Give the Little Lady a Great Big Hand!

Body language expresses your newfound confidence in the long shots, but let's get back to your Close-ups. Right along with facial expressions, your hands are continually expressing (and revealing!) your emotions, your intentions and your inner sense of self. In Chapter 8 we learned the power of that unspoken dialogue that is expressed through our eyes. The language of hand gestures is another unspoken language that we all use and understand.

Just as eyes can project either alluring or assertive messages, so hand gestures can underline or undermine the intentions expressed by your face and your words.

Feminine, seductive hand gestures. These are slow, languid movements; circular, rounded gestures with fingers curved and separated, wrists relaxed, the palm open and exposed. Playing with a bracelet or necklace, twisting or playing with jewelry, scarves or belts, twisting a curl, pushing hair back from the face or curling it behind on ear are all alluring hand gestures.

Assertive hand gestures. Assertive gestures are made with fingers straight and together, the palm down or otherwise concealed. They are straight, choppy, short movements with a stiff wrist. According to Judy Meyers of Meyers and Meyers management consulting firm, two nonassertive hand gestures are fluttering your fingers like jellyfish tentacles, or flapping your hand from your wrist in a fanning motion. Meyers says that both gestures indicate subconscious fears, express a feeling of helplessness, and indicate a lack of control. As with powerful eye language, the best and fastest way to learn appropriate business gestures is to copy someone who uses them well. Look for role models in your real life or watch television figures who hold positions of power and authority. It doesn't matter if your role model is a man because appropriate business gestures express power rather than gender. You won't look masculine using these gestures, you will simply look powerful and give an appropriate background to your business vocabulary.

Age-making gestures. Busy, fussy hands, picking at imaginary lint or smoothing and straightening a collar or sleeve create an impression of age. Clasping your hands together is another age-making image. Check the models in fashion magazines and you'll notice that these vital glamorous creatures are never photographed with their hands together. Instead, their hands are almost always apart, creating a feeling of movement, energy and youth. Clasping your hands placidly and resting them in your lap is another age-making gesture—passive and apathetic.

The language of hand gestures is so eloquent it's easy to see why portrait photographers will often include the hands of a subject in an evocative photograph. And why actresses use their hands to add dimension and emphasis to every emotion. Yes, hand gestures can communicate beyond words, but how your hands *look* will also tell a great deal about your beauty essence.

Tips for Beautiful Hands

Beauty *does* start from within—in that beauty factory of yours that turns a balanced diet into long, strong nails, firm skin, thick, shining hair. But you can't build these beauties on the latest fad diet.

In fact, your fingernails are regular tattletales about your health. According to *Prevention* magazine, "Nails, those horny disposable growths at the ends of your fingers and toes, may be the next rage in the medical world. Researchers are giving them a lot of attention these days. They're discovering that nails grow more slowly in sickness and old age than in youth and good health. Nails are harder in the malnourished than in the well-fed, and there's evidence that deficiencies in iron, zinc and Vitamin E can affect the texture and color of the nails."

What about unflavored gelatin, highly touted as a protein source and a builder of long, beautiful nails? This is just another old wive's tale. Gelatin is not only low in protein compared to other foods, but also the protein it does contain is an incomplete protein, lacking one or more of the eight essential amino acids that the body cannot manufacture itself. Some nutritionists feel that taking large amounts of gelatin can actually produce a dangerous imbalance in essential amino acids. *Protein*, not gelatin, is the magic word. Nails and hair are made mainly of a tough protein called keratin. Being sure that your diet is high in health-building proteins will give your body the building blocks it needs to create beautiful nails.

In addition to diet, what else contributes to nail beauty? Knowledgeable, *consistent* hand care.

Wear rubber gloves! Detergents are the number-one exterior culprit that attacks and weakens your fingernails. Do you really think those tough little bubbles can tell the difference between baked-on *fettuccine Alfredo* and your tender hands and sensitive nails? Moisture is another culprit that negatively affects hand and nail beauty. Too much moisture dries out and chaps the skin of the hands and softens the nails. Rubber gloves are uncomfortable and make your hands clumsy and inefficient? Listen, brain surgeons wear rubber gloves. So can you!

Nail polish is one of the easiest and most effective ways of bolstering the strength of your fingernails. Even the clear kind will add that Close-up finish to your hand beauty, and protect and strengthen your nails, helping them grow longer. Get in the habit of applying a clear coat of polish to the surface and under the tips of your nails every other day.

Beautiful hands not only tell others about your sense of self, but pampered hands have always been a mark of success and privilege. This is why the manicure is always an important part of my TV makeovers. There's nothing like having the hands of a pampered princess to make a woman feel like a true Cinderella.

Hands Up?

You're probably familiar with the simple 7-step technique that constitutes the basic manicure. But, to be sure, let's review it now. (Incidentally, I'm including a couple of little tips that may be new to you.)

Here's the equipment you need:

- Nail polish remover and cotton balls
- Cuticle cream or oil
- Bowl of warm, soapy water
- Nail brush
- Orange stick
- Nippers or nail scissors
- Emery boards
- Hydrogen peroxide (20 percent solution)
- Nail base, polish

MANICURE

1   Remove old polish. Rub remover-soaked squares from base to tip of nail, thus minimizing remover stains.

2   Shape nails with emery board. (Shaping details are in the Close-up Portrait section.) Never file down to the corners. Let your nails grow past the fingertips and then shape the tip.

SPOT ANNOUNCEMENT

DO NOT BEVEL THE NAIL TIP. NAILS ARE FORMED IN LAYERS
AND A BEVELED EDGE CAN CAUSE THE LAYERS TO SEPARATE
AND THE NAIL TO PEEL.

3   Apply cuticle cream or oil and massage into cuticles.

4   Soak fingertips in warm, soapy water to remove oil and to loosen and soften cuticle. Brush cuticle with nail brush to further loosen cuticle. Then dry thoroughly, pushing back cuticle with the towel.

5   Use the orange stick to push back and *gently* lift cuticle. As you work, clean and sterilize the orange stick by dipping it into hydrogen peroxide. This will also bleach the nail tip, keeping it attractively light.

6   Use nail scissors or nippers to remove hangnails or calloused skin. *Do not cut the cuticle.*

7   Apply the nail base and polish to completely dry nails. Stroke from base to tip. Hint: brace fingertips on the edge of a small tray, keep polish bottle on tray in case of spills.

Close-up Portraits

Beautiful, expressive hands are an integral part of a woman's beauty, so it's not surprising that women who have their image in sharp focus have definite ideas on hand care and hand beauty. In my travels crisscrossing the country, I have met many successful and inspiring women who seem to embody the beauty philosophy of each Close-up Portrait. In our walk through the Portrait Gallery today, I'll share with you their unique tips for expressing the beauty essence of your hands and nails.

THE TRULY NATURAL BEAUTY

Tips from a TNB, Sirocco K. of Big Sur.

I think your readers will love this lemon "facial" for your hands. I go out into my garden, pick a fresh lemon right off the tree, then use the juice of one-half of the lemon for the hand facial. (Save the rind for my next tip.) Pour the lemon juice into the palm of your hand, add one-half teaspoon of salt, and massage your hands thoroughly, especially around the cuticle and any callouses you may have. Wash the mixture off. Your hands will be wonderfully soft and silky. This treatment also seems to make them especially receptive to a rich layer of hand cream. I call this lemon facial my natural wonder and I treat my hands every few days.

Here is my *lemon cream for the hands*: use the lemon rind from the above treatment. Fill the "cup" formed by the lemon half with whipping cream. Put this in the fridge overnight. The next morning, you'll see that the cream has become thick and custard-like. Take a teaspoon and mix the softened inner rind into the lemon cream. Apply liberally to the hands. This rich lemony cream softens and silkens the hands remarkably and also gives them a fresh lemon scent.

My Advice: Nail Image for Truly Natural Beauties. Short nails suit your lifestyle and your clothing image, but that doesn't mean that ragged, uneven, unkempt nails will be acceptable. There are several Truly Natural approaches to nail grooming that are in keeping with your overall image. The lemon-juice treatment described above will not only make your hands more attractive but will also bleach nail tips and keep them white. Instead of nail polish, which may seem too artificial for your taste, groom your nails in this way. Use a nail buffing kit to polish them and, if you desire, to impart a soft natural color. These kits are available at beauty supply stores and the cosmetic counters of large department stores. If you're not familiar with this oldie-but-goodie, the kit consists of a chamois-covered buffer and a small pot of nail-polishing cream. The cream is available in tinted form as well as clear. Polishing the nails with the buffer will smooth out any little ridges and impart a delicate luster that is extremely attractive.

CASUAL BEAUTIES

Tips from a CB, Muffie W. of Philadelphia.

Everyone at the club just swears by my pure lanolin treatment for dried-out and calloused hands. I discovered this beauty tip when Feather had dropped her first foal. A product called "Bag Balm" is routinely used to soften and lubricate the mare's milk bag. This pure lanolin product, with its added antiseptic, made my hands look and feel terrific. And it is available at your neighborhood tack shop at a minimum cost for a jug! It does have a slightly medicinal, antiseptic odor, but my friends and I find that this is not unpleasant. In fact, it's somehow reminiscent of early morning rides just hacking across the meadows.

My cousin in Louisville recommends another equestrian product for hardening fingernails. She found that "Hooflex," which had been recommended for her jumper's damaged hoof, was also making her nails stronger and less inclined to break. I bought some and . . . ugh! I hated the odor. But there is a real basis for her enthusiasm. I found a similar cosmetic product available at better stores called Barielle. This pleasantly scented cream, based on the hoof-hardening treatment given to racers at Longchamps, really works to strengthen nails. Believe me, the pleasant scent is worth the price.

My Advice: Hand Care for Casual Beauties. One indispensable hand-care item—whether it be in tack room, tennis gazebo or pool house—is this: hand cream with sunscreen. Yes, I know, hand cream can be a trial for athletic Casual Beauties because the creamy surface makes it difficult to hang onto racket or reins. But that's easy to fix — simply apply a dab of hand cream to the back of one hand, rub vigorously with the back of the other hand. Massage backs of hands together, rubbing in the cream but leaving the palms free of the slippy, slidey product.

Nail Image for Casual Beauties.   There are two nail images that I suggest for Casual Beauties. The first is the most elegantly conservative nail image possible. Keep the nails quite short—the white part would never be longer than a quarter of an inch. Have the nails manicured regularly or groom them yourself, and simply apply a clear polish. You can give this simple elegant look an attractive finish by using a nail-whitening pencil, still available at variety stores or beauty supply houses. Simply moisten the pencil and run it under the surface of the nail for a pure white effect. Bright polish in true red or Bermuda pink is another possibility for you. This will coordinate with your wardrobe colors, but I personally feel that your nails will then have to be worn longer. Bright nail polish on short nails makes fingers look wide and stumpy, not a pretty image.

CONTEMPORARY BEAUTIES

Tips from a Successful CB, Stacey L. of Chicago.

Groomed and pampered hands are an essential element in any power picture. Definitely necessary to take you out of the green eyeshade set and into the realm of powerful privilege. But I find that my nails can be a real trial. Office air is usually so dry, and the dust from the papers I handle adds to the dryness. I keep a tube of ultra-rich hand cream in my desk drawer, and I slip it into my bag along with the key to the executive washroom. After I've washed my hands, I don't dry them thoroughly. Rather, I apply rich hand cream to my still-damp hands and massage this locked-in moisture into my skin. I believe this moisture trick makes a big difference in the effectiveness of any hand cream.

My Advice: Nail Image for Contemporary Beauties. I agree with Stacey. Pampered hands have always been a sign of power, and long nails imply privilege. Somehow we always envision a hand that gestures "off with his head!" as being perfectly groomed, and tipped with long nails. A good guide to nail length that suits *your* hands is this: the white part of your fingernail should be approximately half the length of the pink part. Following this good rule will give you the length that is perfect for your individual nail shape.

Nail shapes go in and out of fashion. The softly rounded oval-shaped nail is the most conservative, fashionably speaking; a straight-sided nail with a slightly rounded top is the most current contemporary look. Do wear nail polish, Contemporary Beauties. Fluorescent lights make hands as well as faces look pale and fragile. Hardly the capable image that says "Don't worry, J.B. I can take the reins until you're feeling better." Take color cues from your lipstick shades, and keep a bottle in your desk for touch-ups.

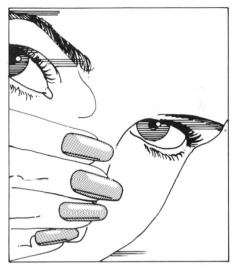

Nail shapes go in and out of fashion—just like clothing styles. Today's look is straight-sided with slightly rounded tip.

DESIGNING BEAUTIES

Tips from a DB, Liz D. of New York.

It's simply essential to realize that nail colors and shapes are part of that total fashion picture. I mean, anybody who's into fashion is aware that those square-shaped long nails that were such attention-getters when Cher made them trendy in the '60s are out of fashion today. The same is true of long, pointed nails. Just check out the hands of the models in your latest *Vogue* or *"W."* Currently fashionable nails seem to be shorter than was chic several seasons ago, but even these shorter nails can break or split. Of course, nail-mending kits work beautifully. But I've found that facial tissue torn into a tiny patch with ragged edges (to sop up the glue) works as well as anything. Use Krazy Glue or nail-mending glue, and apply two layers of these little tissue patches, being sure the glue is dry between applications. Smooth the patch gently with the fine side of an emery board, and then apply ridge filler over the entire nail. This will smooth over the lines of the patched area, and your nail polish will go on smoothly. The split nail may not look perfect, but at least it will pass muster until it grows out. Incidentally, if you've messed up the polish on one nail after perfectly manicuring the other nine, save their polished perfection by using a Q-Tip saturated with polish remover on that one offender. This will keep the remover off the perfect ones.

My Advice: Nail Image for Designing Beauties. DBs are as adept at shaping and contouring their nails to flatter their hands as they are at sculpturing their faces to create the most flattering facial proportions. Here are some guidelines. The most flattering shape for most hands is a straight-sided nail with a slightly rounded tip. This shape also adds to nail strength by keeping the sides straight rather than filing them in and thus weakening them. Still, if you have wide, short-bodied nails, better to wear them shorter and file them into an oval shape.

Short, wide-bodied nails or fan-shaped nails can be contoured with nail polish into a longer and narrower shape. It's simple—just don't apply nail polish to the very edge of the nail base. Very narrow nails, with a small pink area, look wider and more beautifully proportioned if you do not wear them too long because added length accentuates too-narrow nails. A medium length filed in a rounded-squared shape will make this small nail look larger. Short stubby fingers and wide nails look longer and more graceful if you wear pale polish that visually extends the length of your fingers, clear to the very nail tip.

THE ALLURING BEAUTY

Tips from a Glamorous AB, Cheri M. of Beverly Hills.

You never know when someone will want to kiss your hand. For that reason, I always use a hand lotion chosen from my favorite fragrance line. This way the cloud of Shalimar or Joy or Chloe goes from the top of my head to the tip of my toes because, yes, I apply this fragrant hand lotion to my feet too. Believe me, pretty feet are *so* sexy—I never forget the importance of those other ten nails. Pedicures are a must on my beauty schedule. And just for the fun of it I sometimes apply an absolutely *wild* shade of polish to my toenails: glitzy orange or gold or something so crazy that I'd never wear it on my hands. Like seductive or playful lingerie, this becomes another one of those "it's our secret" tantalizers.

My Advice: Nail Image for Alluring Beauties.   Every Alluring Beauty has long, ultra-feminine nails. They are a definite turn-on, implying a hint of animal passion, from pussycat to wildcat. The only possible shape for long, sexy nails is straight-sided with a slightly rounded top. As in all elements of the Alluring Beauty's image, sex appeal must be tempered by taste and subtlety: long nails with bright red polish are definitely sexy, but long, red, *very pointed* nails are definitely a case of overkill.

Nail polish colors for the Alluring Beauty follow the same color themes as Alluring lipstick plans. Bright red and bright pink polishes are both possibilities. A different kind of ultra-feminine image is expressed by the long pale nail. Tan hands with pale opaque beige polish creates a very California look. And polishes in a multihued opaline iridescence will give you moon-goddess hands. The opalescent polish replaces the old outmoded pearlized types that were once so favored by Alluring Beauties everywhere.

Yes, every Alluring Beauty has long, feminine nails, whether they are her own or created by a number of magical techniques known to top manicurists. Long nails can be created through the use of acrylics, nail tips or nail wraps. Here's a rundown of each type including the pros and cons of each nail-lengthening treatment.

● Acrylic nails are formed of dental acrylic, brushed over your regular nail, and onto a paper form which allows the manicurist to extend the acrylic tip to a glamorous length. Acrylic nails look natural, are not fragile and, if you are faithful about getting the ten-day fill-in repairs, will last indefinitely. It's not a good idea to leave the acrylic covering on, month in and month out. Your own nail will grow out underneath the acrylic, but it will tend to become very soft. Therefore, you should have your manicurist remove the acrylic nail every three or four months and allow your own nails to "breathe" and return to their natural state. Incidentally, acrylic nails must be removed *carefully*. Your manicurist will have you soak your fingers in nail polish remover, then she'll carefully chip away at the acrylic covering until it comes off.

● An alternate to acrylic is the nail wrap, an elaborate technique rivaling origami paper folding. It employs glue-soaked tissue paper or silk fabric carefully wrapped and folded around the long tip of your own nail. Layers of glue and polish further reinforce and strengthen the paper-wrapped tip. I personally feel this technique is best for overall nail health. Month in and month out, your paper-wrapped nails maintain their natural texture, and problems with fungus (fairly common under acrylic nails) or other infections are minimized by the nail-wrap method. Unfortunately, it takes much longer to achieve, and it's difficult to find a real artist at this demanding skill. Also, nail wraps are more fragile than acrylics. They must be totally redone every ten days to two weeks. Nail tips can be a combination of tip plus acrylic covering or tip plus nail wrap. Either approach can be totally successful given the pros and cons of the auxiliary technique.

Fashion magazines and beauty books are filled with information on how you can do these elaborate nail techniques yourself. Good luck! Frankly, I believe that beautiful nails via the sophisticated techniques I've just been describing are only possible with a manicurist and a talented one at that. The cost, thirty to fifty dollars for a complete set of nail extensions, and three to five dollars for repairs, can make long alluring nails an impossible dream. Still, Alluring Beauties everywhere seem to find room for this expenditure in their budgets.

THE AGELESS BEAUTY

Tips from an Elegant AB, Linda Sue T. of Dallas.

If you can't beat 'em, join 'em. That's been my solution to those unsightly brown spots on the backs of my hands. I got tired of using bleaching cream which wasn't very effective. Instead, I decided to apply tanning gel, the kind that gives you a lasting tan without the sun, over the backs of my hands and on my forearms. The brown spots blend into my newly tan hands, and I love the healthy look this gives me. So much more vital than pale, fragile, possibly blue-veined hands.

Of course, I faithfully use sunscreen too. I mean, I don't acquire this look with a bona fide tan. I realize that those brown spots are really sunspots and are caused by extended exposure to ultraviolet light. Incidentally, light bright nail polish in golden colors ranging from coral to apricot is wonderfully flattering to my newly tanned hands and to my emeralds, too.

My Advice: Nail Image for Ageless Beauties. Check out nail images for Designing and Alluring Beauties. Long glamorous nails will make ageless hands look terrific. And, now that you've earned a bit of self-indulgence, perhaps longer alluring nail lengths via acrylics or wraps will fit into your life style. Be aware that, as with every element in the Ageless image, outmoded nail shapes and nail polish colors can make mature hands look matronly instead of ageless.

What's out: safe, traditional oval-shaped nails will make mature hands look older. The straight-sided nail with a slightly rounded top is a current look that makes hands look ageless. Pointy nails are also agemakers, hopelessly dated and, worst of all, making you look like you're trying too hard to fit into a dated Alluring image. Reread the section on Designing nails and be aware that nail polish colors make a fashion statement right along with hemlines. Safe, muted moss-rose nail polish colors are impossibly matronly. Any blue-toned polish will call attention to veins and make mature hands look fragile and old. Bright polish tones in light bright red, coral, peach, apricot are super-flattering. Or choose dramatic pales—moon shades, beiges. Or vivid true pinks.

Another key to ageless hands is exercise. Like every single part of our bodies, hands respond miraculously to exercise and the reward is firm, youthful skin combined with grace and agility. Here are two easy exercises that can be performed almost anytime you are alone.

The Grabber: Extend arms straight out in front of you with all ten fingers stretched wide. Now bend elbows and pull hands back toward your body, at the same time pulling fingers in to form a tight fist. Now extend arms straight out and stick fingers out. Grab in, clenching fingers tightly, stretch out, stretching fingers wide. Alternate this stretching/clenching movement. What does this do? Just try it for ten counts. You'll see!

The Chopin: As the name implies, you simply pretend that you are playing a complicated piano cadenza, moving all ten fingers rapidly over an imaginary keyboard. Continue for a count of ten to start with; build up to twenty, then fifty.

Your hands tell you that these two exercises really give the tiny muscles and tendons of your hands a workout. Your eyes will tell you that exercise, faithfully performed, benefits your hands as it does every part of your body.

Day 9 — Beauty Essence Workout: Create Your Own Magic Mirror

I learned about the Magic Mirror trick several years ago when I was interviewing one of England's most successful stage actresses. We met backstage in her dressing room, and while we talked she sat in front of a standard makeup table ringed with bare bulbs. As she completed removing her stage makeup and looked at her bare face in that uncompromising light, she said, "M'gawd, I look bloody awful, don't I? If I believed this mirror, I'd pack it in—never leave this dressing room. Thank heaven, I've got my Magic Mirror. You have no idea how it helps with that terrifying Grand Entrance when one sweeps out on stage, alone except for one's face! But my Magic Mirror gives me that little jolt of confidence that I need."

She gestured toward the dressing room door and I noticed a mirror hanging beside it. There was a slight peachy tint to the glass, and an ordinary clip light had been rigged just at the top of the mirror. "Notice the lighting and the color of the mirror? That peachy tint does wonders for the complexion, and the key light is placed to give me the most flattering image possible. That's the last reflection I see of myself before I go out to charm and enchant that audience. And my Magic Mirror reflection makes me feel capable of doing just that. I can't tell you how many times my Magic Mirror has given me that little morale boost I need to give a really good performance, to relax, forget about myself, and just express my best." She went on to explain that she had arranged to have the same mirror set-up in her Mayfair apartment and her country home. "Whenever I leave my apartment or my dressing room, I look at myself in my Magic Mirror—the one that shows me in a most flattering reflection. Because, after all, *that's real too.*"

I urge you to set up a Magic Mirror somewhere in your home—preferably by the door you use most often. This is your checkpoint, the final reflection you see before you go out to meet your world.

What kind of lighting will you need to make your Magic Mirror most effective? I asked photographer Bill Santos, who recommended soft, diffused light, the very same kind he uses to get terrific fashion pictures. "A simple and inexpensive light that I've been using here in the studio is available at hardware stores. It's a large frosted globe, about four inches in diameter, that just screws into any socket; no special fixture is necessary. It looks attractive and creates a wonderful light source." Other bulbs, to be used in hanging lamp or wall fixtures, should have soft white, pink or amber tones. Or you might choose a light fixture with a warm-toned shade. Santos suggests using a "key" light: a single light source as close to eye level as possible. Or use two lights, again at eye level, one on either side of your Magic Mirror.

Does this seem to be an elaborate scheme, terribly self-engrossed and vain? I'm simply advocating that this mirror image reflect you *at your very best*! Flattery is good for you. Like a generous friend, your Magic Mirror gives you a compliment as you leave the security of home to face the demands of the world.

Your makeup mirror is a friend, too, but it's blunt and straightforward. On some gray morning when you know you're stepping out to meet big challenges, it's very comforting and confidence-building to have a second opinion, the opinion of your Magic Mirror.

Thirteen

DAY TEN

Photo Finish!
Your "After" Picture

It may come as a shock to you, but in the final day of your Close-up Makeover program, I'm going to show you how to have your picture taken! You may be inclined to skip this step and forget about having a formal "after" picture of the new You taken by a professional photographer, but you *must* go through with it. This last step is a very important part of your Close-up Makeover.

As you'll see, it has far-reaching effects, not only helping you to maintain your Close-up Makeover, but also adding to that strengthened self-confidence that is such an integral part of my makeover process. You'll receive bonuses far beyond your "after" picture. You'll feel relaxed and comfortable on vacations, at parties, weddings, christenings, and bar mitzvahs when some camera bug calls out, "Say cheese!" And professionally, confidence before the candid camera will save you from embarrassment and nervousness when the company photographer stalks the meeting rooms at that next business conference, snapping photos for the company newsletter. You'll look professional because you've prepared your professional photo image.

The Right Makeup for Your "After" Picture

Makeup for your "after" photo session will be slightly different from your regular Close-up makeup plan. As any professional photographer will tell you, the right makeup is a vital element in creating the best photographic results, a means of retouching *before* the picture is ever taken.

So an important part of your preparation involves a review of all your Close-up makeup techniques, especially the section on sculpturing. The procedure and makeup principles for your "after" photo are almost the same. But there are some differences.

For photography, the most important makeup item is the base. Whether in color or black and white, a smoothly applied base creates the illusion of flawless skin, and is the perfect foundation for corrective sculpturing. The makeup base that you wear every day should be right with these exceptions:

1 If you are a fair-skinned blonde you will photograph better with a foundation makeup that is at least two shades darker than your regular base. This color depth will create pleasing contrast between your fair hair and pale skin. If you have gray or silver hair, the same concept applies.

2 If you are a brunette with medium to olive skin you'll photograph best with makeup base that is one shade lighter than your daytime makeup.

3 If your skin is dark brown, use the same base that you use for street wear.

Note: Photographically, anytime you use a makeup base that does not match your skin exactly, be sure to apply it to your neck and ears as well. Also, since you may wish to have your hands in the picture, it's a good idea to apply makeup to the backs of your hands too. Blend carefully with a makeup sponge.

As we've already learned, sculpturing can be used effectively in your daytime makeup plan but it has to be extremely subtle in that context. For black-and-white film, however, you can expect much more dramatic results because the shades you use will be much stronger in contrast—the dark, minimizing creams and powders can be two shades darker than your base, and your highlighting items can be two or three shades lighter.

Follow the same corrective plan you've already developed, but your shadows and highlights can be more dramatic and obvious. This does not mean that your application can be slap-dash. In fact, because the camera magnifies every detail, it is important to blend and blend with your makeup sponge and brushes, being sure that no line of demarcation exists wherever you have applied sculpture cream and powder.

Because blushers and face color will create a dark shadow on black and white film, cream rouge and face color should not be used at all. Now is the time to use powder blush to accent or create cheekbone hollows. Use bronze, amber or brick-toned powder blush for this. Then dust just a bit of very pale pink blush on the "apples" of your cheeks as a morale booster.

Black-and-white film intensifies red shades—a true red blouse, for example, will photograph black. So you should choose lighter lipstick shades, no matter what you are currently wearing in real life. The best lip color choices are bright corals, poppy reds and true reds. Avoid colors with blue undertones, deep reds, brick and brown shades.

Eye makeup for black-and-white photography is based on brown eye shadow in shades ranging from taupe to mushroom to rosy brick, and on black eyeliner and mascara.

Will your photo-finish makeup plan have a matte or luster finish? The choice is yours, based on your Close-up Portrait image. But you should use more powder for camera makeup than you would ever use for daily wear because the camera accents any shine and oiliness on the skin. Use a translucent colorless powder for this—your baby talc will even work, in a pinch!

How to Be Photogenic

Do you think models and actresses just automatically know how to turn their best side to the camera, how to flash that perfect smile, how to create the magnetic glance that will push the Pepsi sales over this month's quota?

Listen, they practice and practice and rehearse for many hours before the mirror to perfect that dynamite smile, that delicious glance, that evocative body stance. Every professional in front of a camera has a repertoire of smiles, expressions and poses carefully developed away from the camera. *Yes,* I am suggesting that you lock yourself in the bathroom and spend a few minutes practicing your smile and facial expression. You'll be using a specific, analytical method that will give you more awareness of your own face, your own best features, and you'll have much more self-confidence when you're in front of the camera.

Okay. Let's rehearse. Here are your props—bathroom or dressing-table mirror and a nonmagnifying hand mirror. By now, after working with my Objectivision techniques, you know a lot about your face—its pluses and minuses. Using the double-mirror technique (Objectivision #2), let's review your analysis of your face.

1 Front view. How symmetrical or asymmetrical is your face? If feature placement makes your face extremely asymmetrical, avoid any "straight-on" photos. Even when the photographer says, "Okay, now look straight into the camera," you'll "cheat" a bit, turning your face imperceptibly so that your best side is toward it. Even angling your face one-half to three-quarters of an inch can make an amazing difference in the camera image that will be recorded.

2 Using the double-mirror method, turn your face slowly from side to side and decide which you like better. Now you know which side of your face is more photogenic. And you have the answer to why some of your photos are pleasing, while others seem so unflattering. Whenever possible, in studio photos or candid shots, turn this side toward the camera. And don't keep this knowledge a secret! Tell your photographer which side you prefer.

3 Your eyes, always your most expressive feature, need a little guidance in telegraphing their message through the camera and onto film. When photographed, the natural eye contour tends to create a sleepy-eyed look that is not photogenic. Here is an exercise that is a staple in the model/actress's bag of tricks.

Looking directly into your hand mirror, note how the natural position of your upper eyelid partially covers the upper part of your eye. Now, consciously try to lift your upper eyelid to make your eyes appear larger. No—that's not quite the idea. Opening your eyes wide in a "Wow! Little Me on Candid Camera?!" expression is too much of a good thing. Start again and try to raise that upper eyelid just a fraction of an inch. Relax. Now, try again—just consciously think of lifting the eyelid. See how your eyes look larger, younger, more beautiful? See why models take the time to perfect this little lids-up trick?

Practice not only makes perfect, it makes possible. You *can* learn to control this muscle. Work on it, for better pictures every time.

4 Next, look directly at your reflection in the large mirror and practice smiles. A little smile, a medium smile, a great *big* smile. Do you like what you see? Right away, you'll probably notice that the Great Big Smile—the one Uncle Ed is always urging you to display at family picnics—is the least flattering, creating heavy smile lines, scrunching up your eyes, and possibly showing more gums than ivory. Okay, turn down the volume of that smile—and I mean just that. Smile broadly, and then think of turning down the volume on your stereo—slowly, imperceptibly, you can still have a warm smile, but one that is not so reminiscent of Halloween!

Now, experiment a little bit. Close your mouth so that your teeth are together in a soft bite. Smile. How does that look? Next, open your mouth slightly so teeth aren't touching. Smile. What do you think? Finally, open your mouth about one inch—that's a pretty wide open, Marilyn Monroe smile. Do you like it? Another trick, one that will tighten the area under your chin, is to place the tip of your tongue on the roof of your mouth, and smile, smile, smile.

Do you still feel self-conscious about being so analytical, so self-engrossed with your image? There's no need to. This self-analysis can give you a lot of confidence in front of the camera.

Finding the Perfect Photographer

Every Hollywood star has her favorite director, the one who is able to inspire her most meaningful, most dynamic performance. In the same way, you and your photographer will work together like the star and the director to achieve an "after" picture that will be an award winner. That's why it's so important now to shop carefully for the perfect photographer for you.

What about recruiting talented husbands/lovers/friends to take your "afterpix"? It's okay *as a last resort,* but it's much better if you can afford an outsider. Your "after" picture is special, so I must recommend a photo session with a pro as the ideal culmination of your 10-Day Close-up Makeover.

Every city of any size has hundreds and hundreds of photographers, all of whom are very competent and capable technically. But you want to find the one who will work with you to create your Close-up Portrait, the "after" picture that expresses the real You.

Assuming that he has all the technical abilities to deliver a professional portrait, there are really only two elements to consider in choosing a photographer: personality and working style.

PERSONALITY

This element is very important to you because it determines how you're going to respond in front of the camera. A compatible photographer is going to cue into *your* personality, to help you reveal your inner essence. When you shop for the right one, share with him the details of your Close-up Makeover, the elements of your Close-up Portrait, and exactly the final result that you want.

WORKING STYLE

Some commercial photographers and most professional photographers prefer to work in the studio, in a more formalized atmosphere with lots of lights and the ability to control the environment totally. Others do their best work outdoors. This approach represents a freer, more spontaneous way of working, which has its advantages, but the control over the light is not quite so absolute. Your Close-up Portrait can help you to decide which style is right for you.

The Photo Session

Let's block out the scene for a typical photo session so you will know exactly what to expect and be comfortable with it. Understanding the working challenges that your photographer faces will help you cooperate with him and respond effectively to his directions.

You arrive at the photo studio and chat with your photographer for a few minutes. He'll look at the various costumes you brought and you'll discuss what to wear, how you will do your hair. Perhaps he'll give you a few suggestions on your makeup or, in some studios, there may be a makeup person there to help you. (By now, of course, you don't need the extra help!)

During this initial discussion the photographer is looking at you as you talk, analyzing your face, mentally clicking off good and bad camera angles. Obviously, it's also a chance to break the ice. I can't stress this often enough: a really wonderful photograph is the result of you and the photographer working together.

Once you've changed into your outfit for the photo, the photographer will seat you in front of the camera. At this point he begins doing all kinds of technical things. He goes behind the camera and looks at you, he moves around and fiddles with lights, he gets his light meter and brings it up to the tip of your nose and squints his eyes up and looks at some mysterious dials on the light meter and looks at you and perhaps hums a little tune and walks around and fiddles with the lights again. You see a man happy in his element.

But are you happy? You've psyched yourself up all morning to have these very important pictures taken and now, suddenly, every hangup you've ever had about your looks starts appearing on the screen of your mind with depressing clarity.

"I have a funny smile." "My nose is too long." "My ears stand out." Stop! Now is the time to take charge of your inner dialogue. In these few minutes when all of the photographer's attention is on the technical aspect of the shoot, you must do *your* work.

Mentally review the exercises that we have completed in former lessons: the eye contact, the technique of projecting your dynamic energy, the facial expressions that you have practiced until they have become natural. During this preparation period, while you may be chatting with the photographer and possibly getting rid of a little nervous energy, on some level of your personality you are conserving your energy, holding it in check, waiting to project all of that dynamic vitality into the camera lens. Can you do it? Of course—just hold back a bit of your personality, keep it hot, alive, electric, to project into the camera's lens.

All the great models and actresses know this technique of zapping the camera. A friend of mine who recently worked with Catherine Deneuve on a TV commercial described the phenomenon:

> She came into the studio looking much smaller than I imagined—pale, fragile, and really not a woman that you would look at twice if you saw her on the street. After she had applied her camera makeup and had her hair done, she was beginning to look more like the superstar that she is. Still, I found myself wondering: what's all the fuss about? But then when Deneuve was in front of the camera and the filming actually started, it was like seeing a bolt of electricity emerge from this dynamic blonde and project right into the camera's lens. That's star quality. Unmistakably.

A final bit of advice. One of the biggest problems that amateurs have in working in front of the camera is that they are unsure of how to follow the photographer's directions. The following tips will help you work with your photographer/director like a real pro:

Listen.   When your photographer asks you to move your head to the left, he will mean to *your* left. When he directs you to lean more to the right, to cross your leg, to turn your body more toward the camera, listen to his directions. I have observed so many times that amateurs in front of the camera simply do not listen to the directions they are given. This is often the result of nervousness and stagefright, but it may also stem from inattention. Listen carefully to the directions your photographer gives you and follow them.

Movement.   When your photographer asks you to "turn to the left" or "move your head to the right," he usually means a *slight* turn. Get in the habit of moving slowly and gradually as you follow the photographer's directions. Usually he wants just a slight change in your pose, one that will reflect the most flattering camera angle. Quick, expansive movements will shatter the camera image he's working with and will destroy the easy, relaxed mood that is necessary for both of you to produce the best photograph.

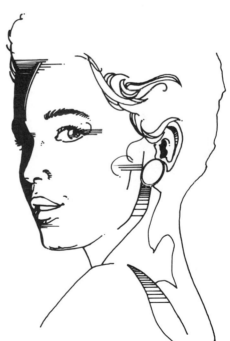

Your photographer will direct your line of vision to create dramatic impact in your "after" picture.

Eyes.   Because your eyes are the focal point of every effective photograph, your photographer will often direct your line of vision to create an effect that he is looking for. "Turn your eyes to the left, please" means simply that . . . very slowly, move your eyes toward your left shoulder. *That does not mean turn your head to the left.* Become accustomed to moving your eyes and not your head when asked to direct your line of vision.

Finally, remember that whatever is closest to the camera lens will photograph larger; what is farthest from the camera lens will photograph smaller. A perfect example to illustrate this point is the standard chest-out, buns-back pose of the Playboy bunny. With this pose, chests look larger, hips look smaller. Usually you will place the weight of your body away from the camera, but occasionally the photographer will ask you to lean forward or to shift your weight in some manner. Again, *listen* to the directions he gives you and be aware that hips, shoulders, head, arms and hands will all photograph slightly differently depending on their proximity to the camera.

The photographer is now ready to start photographing you. Lights, camera, action. At this point, like any skilled director, he will begin to talk to you—to interact with you in order to elicit that energy, that electricity, that magnetism. Now you should respond to his comments and turn on for the camera.

There are as many working styles as there are photographers. Some stand quietly behind the camera, but a newer approach is the active, candid technique. Don't be surprised if your photographer starts moving around the set, his camera on motor-drive . . . clicking, clicking, clicking . . . taking multi-poses of you, all the time keeping up a litany of "fabulous," "you look marvelous," "gorgeous, babe," "that's terrific." What he's doing is keeping the energy flow going. He's praising you, flattering you to continue to get the dynamic response that he sees through the camera lens. And it's important that you do respond to his direction. *But always respond within the character of the Close-up Portrait you have chosen to express.* Continue to be aware of the inner mood you have created.

Day 10—Beauty Essence Workout: How to Use Your "After" Photo to Direct Your Image-ination

The "after" picture is a reward for you, concrete evidence that you have progressed through your 10-Day Close-up Makeover and have *actively* taken charge of your looks to bring about positive change.

But it is more than a record of accomplishment. Your "after" picture is an invaluable tool in helping you to generate *continuing,* positive changes in your looks—and in your life.

Movie stars, billionaires, top executives, people of accomplishment in all walks of life usually have pictures of themselves in their office or dressing room. I've observed this phenomenon almost without exception among the many famous and successful people I've met in my work. They all seem to cherish a visual record of their accomplishment through publicity photos and flattering portraits, candid pix of awards, and casual photos with the even more famous ("Yeah, that's me and Kissinger. He really is a teddy bear.") The unthinking and possibly envious person misinterprets this display, judging it to be vanity, pure and simple. But wait. There is a valuable success lesson to be learned here. These personal and flattering photo records of accomplishment are a powerful means of reinforcing image-ination—beauty, confidence, power, success—the image-ination continues to create the reality of these positive photo images. Yes, imaging one's success is a well-known tool among people of great accomplishment. And that's why you are going to keep your "after" picture in a place where you can see it daily.

Do not put it away (in a "memory" book?) after you have given one to the man in your life, your mother, and maybe to a best friend. No. Keep a copy of your "after" picture in a place where you can see it often. Use this record of your accomplishment to fire *your* image-ination. Incidentally, I use the term "after picture" but there's no reason why you can't have many "after" pictures to motivate you, to guide you and to stimulate you to continue this thrilling adventure in self-development.

I urge you to get in the habit of having photographs taken whenever the opportunity presents itself. Talented amateurs will love to snap photos of the new You, so be a willing and enthusiastic model. If, several months from now, you feel you can budget another photo session, do so. In other words, don't get stuck in that "after" picture feeling that it is the pinnacle of your life's accomplishment. Your image, like your life, will not remain static and your "after" picture(s) will be a continuing inspiration. Change is the essence of life. Use your "after" picture and subsequent photos to give yourself concrete, visible evidence of the infinite possibilities that are within you! Your "after" picture(s) will be a continuing inspiration.

Fourteen

Your Close-up Makeover and Your Leading Man

There's a new woman in his life—you! In this chapter we'll be examining your man's possible reactions to your Close-up Makeover. A man typically exhibits one of two reactions to his partner's makeover. Either he is thrilled or he is threatened—in either case, he is thrown. If your Leading Man is thrilled, what more could you hope for? *Enjoy.* You have gotten the reaction that every woman hopes for when she undertakes a makeover, and you have provided your loved one with what he has always wanted—*variety!* According to clinical psychologist Carol Altman, variety is what men want most in marriage. And she is not the only expert in the field of marriage counseling and sex therapy to say so. Everyone from Dr. Joyce Brothers to Shere Hite has emphasized the importance of the "harem fantasy" in male sexuality.

I won't promise that using your Close-up Makeover to satisfy your Leading Man's craving for variety will make him a totally happy and contented creature. But more likely, he will be bemused, intrigued and fascinated, which sounds like a lot more fun than the fully domesticated, pipe-and-slippers breed of male. For example, here are stories that two newly madeover women have passed along to me:

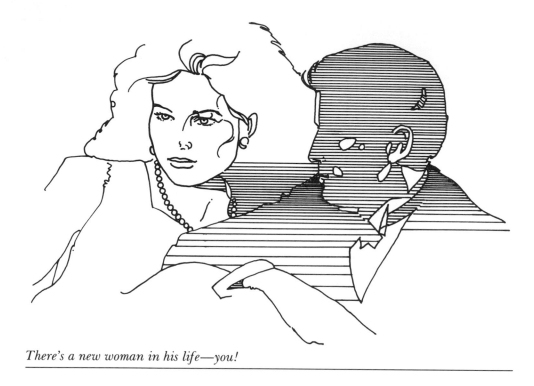

There's a new woman in his life—you!

● Elizabeth, blushing prettily and looking rather smug, reported that her husband (a man of few words) took one look at her and exclaimed "I can't wait to get this beautiful blonde into bed!"

● Helene's husband was the shy type. She told me that he studied her closely all through dinner, then finally whispered, "I feel as though I'm having an affair with a new woman."

These comments again confirm the truth inherent in that old adage, "Woman's greatest asset is man's imagination." The brain is indeed the first erogenous zone. Your Close-up Makeover can help you use *his* imagination to *your* advantage.

If He Feels Threatened . . .

Sometimes the results of my Close-up Makeover are so spectacular that a husband or boyfriend becomes frightened and jealous. And we can hardly blame him—will he lose the now-stunning companion of his life to an oil tycoon or a movie star? The man is *worried*. If this applies to your Leading Man, the best approach is to immediately administer massive doses of flattery, attention and TLC. Once he is thoroughly reassured that he will not lose you, he should respond to the enormous ego boost that you, the beautiful, confident woman in his life, provide. So bolster his ego and give him confidence that your relationship remains on solid ground—he'll soon start to enjoy the rewards of life with the new you.

Here is another tactic that has often proved effective in dealing with a Leading Man who feels threatened by your transformation. It must be handled with the utmost delicacy and discretion, however. Take the opportunity to very gently and cleverly lead him toward a makeover of his own!

It has been my experience that a great many men are fascinated with the idea of improving their appearance—it's just that they don't have the slightest idea of what to do or how to go about it. You might subtly try to feel him out on the subject of hair color, a new hairstyle, losing some weight, using a face bronzer or other skin-care products, or even having cosmetic surgery. All of the options listed above are just as applicable to the young man as to the men of "distinguished" age.

For heaven's sake, *don't* suggest all of these things to him at once. Your strategy is to let him know that you are there to help him make the most of his looks, now that you have successfully improved yours. If you go about it carefully, the results can be extremely rewarding. I've seen it happen: becoming the Beautiful People together can be a great new form of togetherness.

Your Makeover and the Leading Men in Your Life

We have been talking about marriages or long-term relationships, but what if you are footloose, fancy-free and shopping? What if you have not yet begun to shop? All the more reason, then, to acquaint yourself with what men find irresistible in a woman. Numerous experts (everyone from Helen Gurley Brown to Zsa Zsa Gabor) have told us that the single most attractive quality a woman can possess is *confidence*—the kind of self-confidence that shows the world you are comfortable with yourself as a woman and are at ease with both the inner and the outer you.

If you are single and dating, there is absolutely nothing that will give you more social confidence than knowing that you are your most attractive, pulled-together self. Your Close-up Makeover will bolster your confidence, and thus help you to project the allure of an exciting woman. I urge you to "try on" several of the Close-up Portraits with their various mystiques, and see what type of man each one attracts! Trying on various personas is a chance for you to find out about yourself as well. Psychologists agree that the healthy personality is multifaceted and that it is constantly evolving. You are being unnecessarily inflexible if you feel you have only one hard-and-fast, etched-in-stone personality through which to experience your life. Try on several and see what happens!

To those of you who say, "That's not being honest. I'm tired of having to play games to attract a man," I must reply that I do not agree. Assuming that you have undertaken your Close-up Makeover to please yourself, to release and express the real You, I see no harm in having a little fun with it, in modifying your plan to include the possibility of attracting Mr. Right (or even his cousin, plain old Mr. Wonderful). Recognizing that *you* are the reason you have completed your Close-up Makeover will help you feel more positive toward the "significant others" in your life—husband *or* lover(s).

Fifteen

Why the Stars Are Different

Star Essence — What Is It?

Are the stars *really* different? You bet they are. If you have ever been enchanted by a vision on the silver screen, you *know* they are special. Well, what is it that makes those women so fascinating, so riveting, so mesmerizing? "Easy," you say, "they happen to be gorgeous." I believe that's only part of the story, that the relationship between looks and stardom is not quite that simple and direct. Almost always, the stars themselves have created their own beauty legend.

If you think about most of the great Hollywood stars, you will realize that very few of them were genuine "beauties" in the classic sense. Think of Joan Crawford, Katharine Hepburn, Bette Davis, Ingrid Bergman, Lauren Bacall. Studied objectively, none of these legends represents the "perfect" beauty equation. What they had instead was "Star Essence"—a term I use to describe that special something else that sets the stars apart from the bit players.

I can hear you thinking, "Okay. So maybe they weren't all naturally beautiful, but they had *talent*. It's their talent that made them stars." Sure, talent is necessary. But I know from working in Hollywood that there are many beautiful *talented* artists who aren't stars yet; in fact, most of them don't even have acting jobs. Even when they go hand in hand, beauty and talent do not always add up to Star Essence.

Dreams and Realities

I maintain that there is another quality that contributes to the mysterious allure that characterizes the true stars. They are different because they *know* it. They know they are stars because they have an incontrovertible belief in themselves.

A couple of stories about those two legendary but unrelated Hepburns, Katharine and Audrey, illustrate this aspect of Star Essence. The first is told by Charles Higham in *Kate: The Life of Katharine Hepburn*. In the late 1920s, a very young Katharine was living in a boarding house with a number of other aspiring actors, among them one named George Coulouris. "He [Coulouris] and Kate had a wild effect on each other— sparks flew! After one terrific quarrel, Kate declaimed, 'You can say what you want, but I'll be a star before you're even heard of!'"

The following anecdote about the other famous Hepburn, Audrey, was circulated by venerable press agent Russell Birdwell. Audrey had been brought to Warner Brothers from England where she had enjoyed a modest success in film. She waited and waited, but no script was sent, no role was offered. Finally the call came to report to the studio. Upon arriving she discovered that the part being offered was a walk-on, with perhaps one or two lines.

Most young actresses of the period would have been thrilled to be under contract to Warner's, grateful for even the tiniest part in a Warner's picture. But Audrey Hepburn was not. She marched her petite self up to Mr. Jack Warner and complained about not being cast in a more important role. He replied that that was the only part he had for her, and that she couldn't expect to have star billing. What a nerve she had! She countered with words to this effect: "In my own mind, I *am* a star, and a starring role is the only role I will play."

Well, the rest is history. Audrey's *vision of herself* convinced Warner of her Star Essence. She landed the starring role in *Roman Holiday* opposite Gregory Peck, and her career took off from there. All because she had the courage of her convictions, believed in herself and refused to settle for second best. Now that's an example of Star Essence!

In a more contemporary vein, superstar Cher has said in a recent *Cosmopolitan* interview that she always possessed this kind of certainty—she always knew she would make it big. A survivor of two failed marriages, Cher admits that she was a failure in school (she was an undiagnosed dyslexic), and that she suffered severe skin disorders for years, even after her career got off the ground. Yet she had perfected her "star's autograph" at the age of twelve because, "Somehow, I always thought I'd become something fantastic."

An Inner Awareness

Stars seem to have an inner conviction of their own specialness. But this knowledge, this belief, this conviction alone is not what gives them Star Essence. It is what they *do* with this knowledge that makes them stars. They use it to bring that inner beauty essence into reality, using exactly the same techniques that I have shared with you in your Close-up Makeover. And then, they *project* that reality. They let *others* know that they *know they are special.* Star Essence is the *power of their belief in themselves.*

The strength of a star's vision of herself as special, unique and deserving of the spotlight hypnotizes her audience into believing in her as a star. But the spotlight is not the real goal. The real payoff to stardom is in the opportunity to express to the world one's private vision of one's self as *unique,* as *exciting,* as *special.*

Star Essence and Your Close-up Makeover

We've seen that Star Essence is a magical blend of faith in one's self plus the determination to succeed plus the tools to make that vision a reality. Now, all these anecdotes about stars are undoubtedly interesting. What do they have to do with you? Quite simply, this: your Close-up Makeover has provided you with all the tools—the makeup, the costuming, the script, the rehearsal, and the inspiring direction for *your* starring role, *your* great performance. After all, aren't you the star of your own life? You have spent time, energy and money studying your role and performing the Beauty Essence Workouts. It's time for the payoff. And the big payoff for having faithfully performed your Close-up Makeover is a delicious awareness that you possess your own brand of Star Essence!

Your Close-up Makeover is making a *dynamic* change in your life, because your enhanced image evokes a positive and enthusiastic response from your audience. This in turn further energizes you to make the most of your newfound self-awareness.

Perhaps the words of another Gloria can be helpful here. "Discover the Splendor That Is You" is the ad line for Gloria Vanderbilt's fragrance. That sentence just about sums up everything we have been discussing here. Now that your Close-up Makeover has helped you "discover the splendor that is you," your unique brand of Star Essence, it's time to take things one step further.

Celebrate the Splendor That Is You

Celebrating yourself means reminding yourself of your specialness, reveling in your uniqueness, being good to yourself in big ways and in small ways. You have worked long and hard on your Close-up Makeover. Indulge yourself in the luxuries you deserve—think of them as your reward for having made positive changes in your life. Whether it's relaxing in a milk bath on a rainy afternoon, buying new lingerie, savoring that special imported tea you love, or having a salon manicure—do it!

Treat yourself. Allow yourself some "star trappings," all those little extras that reinforce your belief in your own specialness and make you feel terrific.

Like any experienced director, I know Star Essence when I see it. *And you've got it.* My goal in these pages has been to provide the guidelines that enable you to bring your true image into perfect focus. If I have accomplished that, then my job is complete. I can now step back into the wings as . . .

. . . *YOU* STEP INTO THE SPOTLIGHT. THE MUSIC SWELLS. THE CAMERA ZOOMS IN FOR A CLOSE-UP OF YOU, THE STAR. AS YOU STAND CENTER-STAGE, THUNDEROUS APPLAUSE FILLS YOUR EARS. BRAVISSIMA!

I want to hear about your
Close-up Makeover progress! Write to me

at: CLAIROL
345 Park Avenue
New York, NY 10022

or: P.O. Box 255–827
Sacramento, CA 95865

Acknowledgments

Close-up, more than most books, is the result of the combined efforts of a talented and enthusiastic ensemble. Certainly, my first thank-yous must go to the hundreds of "Close-up Cinderellas," those delightful and inspiring women who *believed* when I said, "Trust me," and put themselves into the hands of my makeover team, to embark on their own exciting Close-up adventures.

I particularly want to acknowledge my debt to my friends and colleagues at Clairol: Jack Shor, Allyn Seidman, Susan Valentine, Karen Fischer, Felicia Gulachenski, and most especially to Phyllis Klein, who is a joy to work with and from whom I continue to learn. Also to Cathi Hunt; to my good friend Barbara Ross, who was there at the beginning; to Fern Kestenbaum; to Mary Frentz; and to Andrea Girard, of ABC Television, always a generous and supportive friend.

Many others have contributed to the successful completion of this book, and to them I extend my deepest appreciation: to Ellen Levine, my literary agent, and her associate Louana Lewis, for their energetic, expert and productive efforts; to Chris Schillig, Associate Publisher at Putnam's, who made the usually traumatic editorial process a constructive and enlightening one; to Sarah Kreps, whose talented and creative input was so invaluable; to Barbara Morgan, who contributed her own form of makeover magic in skillfully typing the manuscript; and to Jeff Hunter, photographer *extraordinaire.*

Finally, my thanks to my friend Jeane Westin, for her initial enthusiasm for the project, for her always constructive criticism, and for her support and encouragement during the long process of writing the book. It is to Jeane that this book is affectionately dedicated.